WINNING
at
LOSING

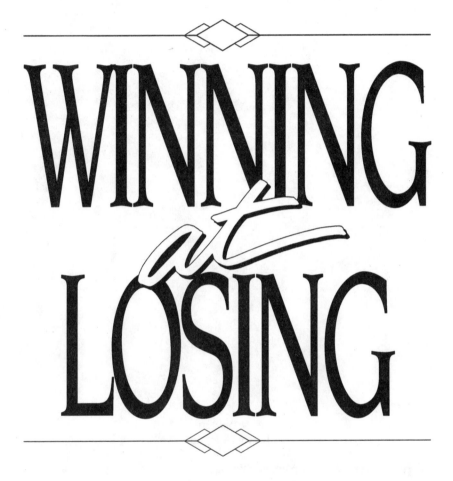

WINNING at LOSING

Jerry B. Jenkins

MOODY PRESS
CHICAGO

ISBN: 0-8024-1737-X

1 3 5 7 9 10 8 6 4 2

Printed in the United States of America

Contents

INTRODUCTION

Waging the War

If you've ever seriously struggled with your weight, you can imagine my fear in allowing my "before and after" pictures on the back cover of this book. We all know that the issue is not losing weight. The issue is keeping it off.

Some say that only 1 in 1,000 who lose more than 100 pounds will keep it off for more than a year. Even the program in which I am involved claims a success rate of just 4 percent. Though I find myself egotistical enough to believe I could be part of that minority, I am also realistic enough not to be over-confident. I am, above all, committed to staying in the battle—with God's help.

I'm going to tell you both stories—the losing and the maintaining—because as a fellow sufferer I know that even though maintenance is the tougher chore, accounts of signifi-cant losses can be intriguing and motivating.

For clarification, let me make this point: I usually try to write as if I am speaking only to you. Yet I don't know if you are fat or thin, succeeding or failing, a fellow struggler or what I refer to as a civilian. Civilians are those who not only do not have weight problems, but they also don't understand them. Most of us enlisted warriors resent people who can eat what they want and not worry.

And so some of what I am writing is for the civilian—for instance, the chapters on what to say and what not to say to a fat person. If you are a civilian, dipping into a book that is by a struggler and for a struggler, my hope is that you will learn how to be a part of the fix and not part of the problem.

More likely, however, you are a fellow combatant in the weight war. My hope and prayer for you is that you will find me sympathetic without excusing and honest without offending. I realize that nearly every diet book you have picked up has made some promise or acknowledged that now, finally, at the end of your rope, you have found the answer. They all say, "You have tried everything else, but now . . ."

There were times, no doubt, when you discovered a book, a program, a plan that really did look like the answer to a lifetime of frustration. But by now you're skeptical of every new approach. You may be coming to this book not with hope, but with resignation.

I'm not going to pretend to tell you things you don't already know. No one is more of an expert than we are about what makes us gain or lose. I'll cover those areas, along with hints and tricks and helps I've learned, so that you can have all that you—and I—know in one handy tool.

The story is here also of *how* I gained my weight in the first place. The *why* is a little more nebulous, which I have found true with every fellow struggler. But putting the details on paper may help me as it helps you, and I encourage you to think through your own history at the same time. The exercise of finally talking about it with people who understand and care is a major step toward success. Otherwise, ours is a most private ordeal.

What I have to offer is that I am finally succeeding after years of failure. It *can* be done, and *you* can do it. But none of us does it alone. Welcome to the part of the journey where the destination finally comes into view.

1

You May Laugh, But It's Not Funny

Fat jokes? I had a million of 'em.

I speak a lot, and I've always known that humor is the great icebreaker. It gives the speaker a chance to calm his nerves while the audience laughs. Once rapport is established, speaking becomes easier.

And I soon learned that self-deprecating humor is the most endearing. If you get up there and make fun of your host or the crowd, it may be funny, but you come off like a smart aleck. An audience has to be in the mood for guys like Don Rickles. Want to connect with a crowd? Tell jokes about yourself.

You've just been introduced as someone with something to say, and naturally your audience wonders if you think you're something special. The ironic, "Wow! I can hardly wait to hear me," might work. Or, "Well, thanks for that introduction, but we all know an expert is merely a guy from out of town." But for someone tipping the scales at between 350 and 380 pounds, there's an easier, more obvious way to endear oneself to an audience.

Comedian Louie Anderson, a fellow struggler, says he always started his act with a joke about his weight because "otherwise people wonder if you know."

When your size is the obvious focus of everyone in the room, you feel obligated to put it in perspective. Some heavy people act overly important or deadly serious. Their weight adds sobriety and import to their message. I, for some reason, felt the need to assure my audience that my weight didn't bother me and so it shouldn't bother them. I was saying, in effect, "I can even make fun of myself."

My opening line, especially in evangelical circles, was a can't-miss. I would ask to be introduced as speaking on "The Lighter Side of [whatever the topic was]." It might be publishing, writing, Sunday school, or sports. As soon as I lumbered to the podium, of course, the snickers began. I would flash my sheepish look and begin, "I know, I know. Asking someone like me to speak on the lighter side is like asking Robert Schuller to speak on the depravity of man."

Depending on the reaction, I might stop there and move into other types of humor or start angling toward my message. Usually, however, the laughter propelled me into a litany of fat-related jokes, all of them true. I share them here for your amusement and instruction, but then I want to tell you what I have come to learn about this type of humor—and in a later chapter the reaction of those who really love me. Make no mistake, the response confirmed that this is funny stuff. But at another level, it's not funny at all.

After the Schuller line, I would continue:

> That's what I like about words: someone who looks like I do can be referred to as a light speaker. Someone who makes people on airplanes religious.
>
> I got on a plane in Chicago recently, and there were only center seats left. I'm telling you, when I move down the aisle, looking for a center seat, people go to prayer.
>
> "Don't do this to me; I've been good!"
>
> I wound up next to a little old man. He didn't scowl at me the way freshly pressed executives do when I settle in. He did, however, wake me with a punch on the shoulder a few minutes after takeoff.
>
> "You don't mind if I punch you when you lean over on me, do you?" he asked.
>
> Let's talk embarrassment. "Not at all," I managed. "I'm sorry."

"Oh, that's all right. It's just that when I'm out in the aisle, no one can get by."

A few years ago I had to take one of those little puddle jumpers, the ones that hold about twenty passengers in seats that can't be more than twelve-inches square.

I was the last one on the plane, and, fortunately, right behind the pilot were two empty seats. One wouldn't have been enough. There wouldn't have been room to turn the other cheek, if you know what I mean. While the copilot was finishing his preflight announcements, the pilot caught sight of my knees in the aisle behind him. He asked his partner, "Is he buckled in?"

The copilot looked at me, wedged in sideways, the toy seat belt buried somewhere, and said, "Hey, he ain't goin' nowhere."

I love it when they inform you that "in the unlikely event of a water landing"—there's a euphemism for you—"you may use your main entrée as a flotation device."

Actually, I find airline food more than palatable as a rule. In fact, when I'm off sugar (usually every Monday), I have trouble passing up the delicious desserts. I don't care for tomatoes and cucumbers, so I take those off my salad and mash them into the dessert. It really doesn't taste too bad.

I got off a plane in London a few years ago, and a business associate picked me up in a little thing he called a car. I didn't know if he was going to strap me on top, or what. He put his wife and five-year-old daughter in the backseat, then opened the passenger side window so I could have one shoulder hanging out, the other in his face.

Meanwhile, his wife was chattering to keep the little girl from saying anything.

"Oh, look, Rachel! Look at the big airplane!"

"We can't see too well from the backseat, can we Mummy?" It's not nice to hit little kids.

Even my own kids give me grief. I was weighing my middle boy, Chad, when he was four. "Forty pounds," I announced.

"Let's see how much you weigh, Dad!"

I stepped on the scales, and we watched the numbers whiz by.

"Hey, Dad! You weigh all of it!"

People on the other end of the age scale are no easier on me. The late evangelist Vance Havner once asked if I had ever tried the garlic sandwich diet.

I said, "*Garlic* sandwiches?!"

"Yeah! You don't lose any weight but you look a little smaller from a distance."

I have to buy my clothes from big and tall men's shops, of course, so when my wife and I noticed an ad—from a standard men's store—for suits up to my size, we just had to check it out. The opportunity for a suit in other than olive drab or khaki does not arise everyday.

"I'd like to see a suit in my size," I told the salesman.

He said, "So would I!"

He threw a tape measure around me—with my wife's assistance. "Well," he said, "we might have one."

I could hardly wait to see it.

Picture this: dark green (at least it wasn't kelly) with orange plaid in four-inch squares.

"I'm gonna look like a ringmaster," I said.

It fit perfectly, as I feared. But when I looked in that three-way mirror (some skinny person's idea) those squares looked like they were moving! My wife and I turned up our noses.

"Let's face it, pal," the salesman said. "No matter what you buy, you're gonna look like a fat guy with a new suit."

"Thank you, Dale Carnegie."

Once, a five-year-old female relative of my wife studied me at the dinner table and announced, "Huh! Little head, big body!"

To which I replied, "Huh! Little body, big mouth!"

That's nothing. A tour guide in Colorado once told our entire group that a Douglas fir with my girth would be ninety feet tall.

A woman friend tells the story of when she was on an industrial strength diet, nibbling at tuna while her family feasted. She served them a delicious, gooey, pecan pie,

and they left one hefty slice, which she put in the refrigerator.

Late in the evening when the kids were asleep and
her husband was upstairs reading in bed, she tidied up
the kitchen and came upon the leftover slice of pie. In a
desperate attempt to keep herself from eating it, she hol-
lered upstairs to her husband. "Honey! You want this last
piece of pie?"

"No thanks, dear," he said. "I don't think I could eat
another thing."

With that she lost all resolve and ate the pie in three
bites.

"Oh, maybe I *will* have it," her husband called out.
"No sense letting it sit around another day!"

"Sorry," she lied. "I just spilled catsup all over it!"

This is the same woman who hid her chocolate bars
in the clothes dryer, and then her teenaged son tossed in
his wet sneakers and turned it on.

Brown Nikes.

I eventually realized that I used fat humor as a shield.

She also claims that one evening for dessert she served
her family a cake she bought at the local grocery. They ate
half of it and encouraged her to at least try a small slice.
She declined.

When they were asleep, she ate the other half. The
next day, while her family was at work and school, she
bought an identical cake, ate half of it, and served the other half for dessert that evening. Her family was amazed at

her resolve--and at how fresh that cake had stayed over-night.

Her most embarrassing moment, however, was when she and her husband and another couple went fishing in a rowboat. Since the fish weren't biting, the couples decided to jump in and frolic.

It was fun until they got back into the boat. Well, three of them got back in. With no pier or dock or anything solid to hold onto, she couldn't get back in the boat. Even with all three helping, there was no way. She had to be towed to shallow water where she could walk to shore.

I'll never forget the time our oldest son, Dallas, told a visitor she was fat.

"I know," she said evenly to our then four-year-old.

Dianna and I came running from different ends of the house.

"You eat too much," he added.

"I know," she said with a frozen smile.

"You need to go on a diet," he said as I scooped him up and transported him from the room.

He got the lecture of his life, which he didn't totally understand. What was wrong, he wondered, with telling the truth? And if my lecture didn't convince him, Dianna's at least reinforced it.

Two weeks later a huge friend of mine joined us for lunch. In midbite, Dallas piped up. "Dad, this time I'm not gonna say anything about anybody bein' fat!"

A few years ago my wife wanted to try parasailing on the beach during a vacation in Acapulco. A speedboat would race up and down the shoreline, lifting the person a hundred feet in the air in a parachute. I asked the man with the boat, "How much?"

He looked us up and down. "For her twenty-five hundred pesos. For you we are closed."

Pretty funny stuff, huh? Depending on the crowd and their mood, by now they were rocking. And what happened later? People wanted to tell me their favorite fat jokes. And because I had told most of these on myself, they knew I'd enjoy being the star of theirs. "Better not get behind you in the buffet line, eh?"

I hid it well, but, strangely, I was not amused. I eventually realized that I used fat humor as a shield. No one wants to be laughed at or made fun of. In other settings, when I had not, in effect, given permission for people to make jokes at my expense, I pointedly ignored them. I wouldn't confront them or say anything, but clearly I didn't laugh and usually pretended not to hear.

Once, in front of a room full of my friends and colleagues, a speaker made a joke about someone having "less work than Jerry Jenkins's workout coach." Another speaker, while I sat forcing a grin at the head table, said that when his kids wanted to swim that afternoon he informed them that they couldn't because "Mr. Jenkins was using the ocean."

Frankly I was gratified when most of the crowd, in both instances, groaned in sympathy. Those jokes were funny, and they might have been socially acceptable had I told them on myself. My line became, "Self-deprecating humor is funniest when it's *self*-deprecating."

Over the years I found myself using my natural bent toward ad-lib humor—even when not telling self-deprecating fat jokes—as a mask. Let me be clear: I wasn't totally aware of this. I have only realized it recently and have come to the conclusion that I was trying (vainly as it turns out) to make a statement: "I take nothing seriously, everything is a joke to me, so let's not worry or even think about this big body, OK?" Those are words no one would ever say, but I believe they evidence part of my motive.

Those who know me well know that I can be every bit as serious as I can be funny. I can be moved. I am an emotional person. And so while speaking I tended to take sharp turns from light to serious. People used to compliment me on how they had never laughed so hard and then been so close to tears. That's not all bad. I still use humor when I speak, and I still use self-deprecating humor. But it is more exaggerated, sillier, not so close to home. It still breaks the ice, and I think people still consider me humorous, but I'm not getting the negative reactions I once did.

Yes, the negatives came, usually second-hand or on evaluation sheets. People who didn't want to offend me still wanted me to know that my fat jokes made them uncomfortable. Sometimes those responses came from people who would write that they had been struggling with their weight for years and felt conspicuous and embarrassed at having the subject raised. Privately I felt bad, but I justified my approach by thinking that I had done the opposite of what they thought. I had taken the spotlight off them and put it on me. I was taking the heat for all the fat people. I could take it. Nothing bothered me. I even believed that myself.

Other times, those negative responses to my fat jokes came from people concerned for their heavy friends. "I was embarrassed for her," they wrote. "I was surprised at your insensitivity." That puzzled me because I thought my being able to take my problem in stride, being unafraid to draw attention to it, showed sensitivity. Only when I thought about my own weariness over everyone else's fat jokes did I get close to understanding what my critics were feeling.

The problem was that for a long time there weren't many critics. Most people enjoy making fun of fat people, and they enjoy fat people making fun of themselves. Overall my evaluations at conferences and banquets were quite high. Humor works. Humor helps people remember. Humor makes pathos more effective. I had a bit of a following, people who not only complimented me but couched it the way I would have: "It's great that you can be so casual about your size. It puts people at ease."

That's where they (and I) were wrong. My fat humor didn't put people in general at ease. It put civilians at ease. It made my fellow strugglers uncomfortable, it hurt those who loved me (as you will see later in my story), and it made me a clown. I was the butt of my own jokes, and I thought that was healthy.

Wrong.

18

2

We All Have Histories

I still use humor when I speak, and I still work in a fat joke occasionally. When people wonder how or why I lost my weight in 1991, I might say I simply got tired of having a driver's license that said, "Photo continued on other side."

Or I might say I was standing alone on a street corner when a cop drove by and told me to break it up. Or that when I was a kid and my friends and I played cowboys and Indians I always had to be the posse. We tried real horses but mine couldn't get his front legs down.

The difference now is that I rarely tell more than one of those, and never more than two. Notice that they are not true, like the ones in the previous chapter. They are silly, less easily identified with. And I usually follow with a serious statement about not wanting to embarrass or offend anyone who is struggling with the same thing I have struggled with.

The fact that I have lost weight and look different than I used to, and that to most people I would no longer be referred to as "fat," doesn't change the facts. Like an alcoholic or a diabetic, I will always be what I am: a compulsive overeater a few thousand calories from disaster.

I put myself in the same category with the overweight people in my audience. I have not separated myself from them just because I lost weight. Rather, I separated myself from them in the past because I pretended not to care. They weren't buying it, and they were right.

The people who loved me said occasionally that they didn't appreciate my weight humor. . . . I recall being uniquely warmed by their concern.

The people who loved me said occasionally that they didn't appreciate my weight humor. They felt I was being too hard on myself. I didn't see it that way, but I recall being uniquely warmed by their concern. They loved me the way I was, and they didn't want anyone—not even me—poking fun.

"I tell the jokes on myself to keep others from doing it," I admitted periodically. But as I've said, the effect was the opposite.

"Let's take a picture of the group," someone would say. "You can be the back row."

To civilians I appeared healthy because I was playing the hand I was dealt. My self-image appeared intact—even to me.

How did I get this way? Every person with a problem has a history. Such can be used as a reason, an excuse, an alibi, or a painful memory. There are times I wish, rashly, that I could point to something in my past to explain my compulsive overeating. Of course, no one wants to have grown up in an alcoholic family or to have had a parent who was obsessive-compulsive or schizophrenic. No one would want to have been abused physically, sexually, or verbally. Yet in the weight control programs I have been involved in over the years, I have heard all those stories.

They are painful, wrenching. I would want to trade places with no one who suffered like that, and yet I felt a strange void. Because there is nothing like that in my history, I could never find a handle on my compulsion. If overeating and being full and becoming fat was a way to hide, a way to put a barrier between you and the world, a warm, fuzzy place where you indulged yourself to mask the pain, then what was my pain? What was I hungry for? What void was I trying to fill?

There were times I thought it would have been handier to be able to say, yes, because this happened to me, I am this way. I have a friend who is obese. His brother is a chain smoker. His sister is an alcoholic. They point to a domineering, dictatorial father who browbeat them into submission until they got out on their own. That knowledge has not helped them overcome their problems, but it has allowed them a handle.

I cannot find any such handle. I was raised in an "Ozzie and Harriet" type home in a friendly little community in a medium-sized, conservative, middle-class Midwestern town. My memories of the community of Oakwood in Kalamazoo, Michigan, are of hardworking, loving parents, lots of friends, a good church, two close older brothers, and a ten-years-later tagalong brother.

My father, a career law enforcement officer, was known for his wisdom, his dignity, his humor, and his sterling character. He didn't swear, he didn't drink, he didn't chase, he wasn't materialistic. He was an unabashed romantic, obviously in love with my mother.

Dad taught Sunday school and sang in the choir. He still does. An ex-Marine and a cop, he didn't have to defend his machismo to anyone. Yet he was never too big to do what needed to be done around the house. I've joked that I resent his example as a man unafraid to scrub a floor, change a diaper, feed a baby, cook a meal, wash the dishes. He showed his love by his actions.

He's not perfect. He had a bit of a temper, though it never resulted in abuse. He might have been more verbal or more physical in his affection, yet, as my eldest brother says, "What else do you call it but love when he was always there when we needed him, digging us out of snowbanks in the middle of the night, lending a hand or a dollar or an ear?"

My dad didn't have a dad. His died when Dad was two years old, and a succession of largely no-account stepfathers were no example. Yet his late mother was strong and resourceful and spiritual. Dad grew up with principles, knew right from wrong, knew that self-discipline was one key to success. But to him success was not measured the way most people measure it. Success was never found in things, in money, or in prestige. It was found in love, in family, in doing the right thing because it's the right thing. It was thinking of others, of being prompt, responsible, dependable. Success meant loving Christ with all your heart.

If there was a chink in my dad's armor when I was growing up, it was that there was no chink. It's taken me years to realize that I had my dad on such a pedestal that I thought I was following a perfect example. That wasn't his fault. He didn't know I felt that way, or he might have been quick to admit faults or remember childhood offenses for me, just so I'd know he was human. If I subconsciously set for myself a goal of being like my dad, without admitting that he had feet of clay, I may have been unrealistic. I may have set myself up for failure. I've always said that if I had half his character I'd be twice the man I am today. I still feel that way, but I don't lay any unreal expectations at his doorstep. He's shown unconditional love and acceptance and pride in all his sons.

To write of my mother is to write of my father as well. They are separate and distinct personalities, of course, but the consistency, the discipline, the reputation, the spirituality seem mirror images to me. Mom would disagree. She would not put herself in Dad's category in those areas. That's what makes their relationship special. Each feels unworthy of the other and grateful to God that He put them together anyway.

Having been raised in a huge, godly family that was largely happy but also knew tragedy, Mom is a fun-loving person. She is more verbal than Dad, more self-revelatory. She is widely gifted with words and music and—like him—is sensitive and caring.

If it sounds as if I have my parents idealized, perhaps I do.

Yet their reputations among friends and relatives is consistent. They are known for their depth, their loyalty, their humility. So, you see, I can't point to some parental dysfunction or trauma.

As for any genetic predisposition to obesity, it's fair to say that though Dad's brothers and sisters were mostly of average size, Mom's—except for her eldest surviving brother—have all struggled with weight. Dad's mother developed diabetes later in life.

My maternal grandfather was always a heavyset man, though at this writing he is in his late nineties and has become thin and frail. My grandmother on my mother's side was insulin dependent most of her life and died of diabetes-related maladies. At least half her offspring developed adult-onset diabetes.

With my weight and my heritage, I was a walking, blood-sugar time bomb. But what might account for the compulsive overeating?

My older brothers and I were born in stair-step fashion in 1946, 1948, and 1949. To many we were like triplets, but I was very aware of the differences. For ten years I was the baby. Jim was the tall, handsome, responsible, mature, voracious reader. Jeff and I were plainer in appearance, but Jeff was an excellent student like Jim and also quite industrious. I was the slob, lazy, into myself, a jabberer, and annoying.

Now, clearly that sounds like a self-image problem, but at the time I was unaware of it. My brothers and I squabbled like most, and as I look back on it, their annoyance with me was justified. The archetypical third child, I was frantic for attention. I was secretly proud of every accomplishment of my brothers, yet I pursued totally different goals. They were in Cub Scouts; I never was. Jim pursued basketball and football, Jeff cross country and track; my sport was baseball. Jim and Jeff became career law enforcement officers. Except for a brief period as an undercover narcotics agent, I pursued journalism.

What do I make of all this? When I pursue the idea of birth order, I have the sense that I'm getting near the edges of my own compulsive behavior. I am not an expert in this area and suspect that psycho-babble is too often related to it. But I do recall a need to prove myself, to live up to something, to show my worthiness. Why? I don't think my brothers really thought I was permanently a no-account. What was I after?

Of all my parents' qualities, one stood out. Some parents have the ability to make each of their children feel like the favorite. Often such children share the humorous secret with their siblings later in life that each was convinced of his position as favored child. Of course, in some families there is clearly a favorite, and everyone knows it. It's the old "Mom always liked you best" routine.

But in our family my parents have been so committed to not showing favoritism that I believe they have convinced us all that we are equal in their eyes. They do it so well because it's true. They are proud of each of us for our own accomplishments, and no matter which of us is praised by someone else, Mom or Dad will work at sharing the spotlight among all the children.

I agree rationally with that approach, find it admirable, and have followed my parents' example with my own children. Yet I sense in myself some subconscious need to retain my parents' approval. Hey, I'm only forty-three!

Such realizations about oneself can be ugly, and I am sorry to say that I have become aware of more of the same. It is said that confession is good for the soul but not for the reputation. My reputation, such as it is, may suffer before I'm through with this exercise. The only reason I want to explore these dark areas is that I am determined to get to the bottom of reasons for an otherwise incomprehensible self-destructive tendency. I have slowly come to the place where I am willing to admit my baseness in this area, in the hope that it might be cathartic to me and instructive to you.

If you share my maddening frustration in trying to get a handle on such a niggling problem, stay with me and privately join the exercise. The experts may judge me an amateur psychologist, but I believe I have discovered some things about myself that shed helpful light on our common dilemma.

3

"Nothing Tastes as Good as Being Thin Feels" Not!

Why do I tell you all this? Who cares about my 1950s TV sitcom parents and my house full of brothers? If you are a fellow struggler, you don't have to ask. It's been my experience that we in the fraternity of the fat (we can call ourselves that in private) do care about each other. We share our stories and admit ruefully our weaknesses in the only setting where everyone else understands and is sympathetic. We want to know of each other's backgrounds, childhoods, marriages, stress, depression, or whatever.

It's everywhere else that we mask our pain. We don't want to provide another reason for civilians to give us "that look" or that shake of the head or, worst of all, that advice. We know our obsession with the past sounds like an excuse. We catch each other rationalizing. I have been through this enough to know when I start putting the blame other than where it belongs. I know my weaknesses and my danger points, so for me to say, "If she hadn't served those chips . . . ," or, "Everybody said I should try the cake . . . ," doesn't get past my baloney filter, let alone anyone else's. Of course, it's always easier to detect everyone else's baloney than our own.

One of the first questions in group therapy or weight control groups is either why you feel you're overweight (strangely not why you feel you overeat, though that is the real issue) or when you first began to have a problem with your weight. Most morbidly obese people (there's a "wake-up call" medical term that will give you pause) trace their weight problems to childhood. But there are the occasional skinnies-through-high-school who develop serious problems later.

I share my own story here only instructionally. You may see things that I have never noticed or understood. I do think the exercise is important, and I apologize in advance for the likelihood that it will seem self-possessed. That is one of our maladies, whether we're gaining, losing, or maintaining.

My first memory of being aware of my body was when I was about seven years old. Childhood pictures show me a typically lean child, not pudgy. I was not quite the string bean that two of my own three boys were in preadolescence, but I recall having little body fat, lanky limbs, and firm torso and chest.

On New Year's Eve the day before 1957 (I had turned seven that September) we prepared to head for festivities at church. I dressed up and stood before the full-length mirror. As was customary, my brothers and I wore similar shirts (amateur psychologists can have fun with that). We had all gotten cowboy boots for Christmas (my brothers' were brown, mine black). Mom had made our cowboy outfits herself. Some of the material we recognized from our old kitchen chairs and thus didn't appreciate until years later when we realized the trouble she had to go to.

Jim was string-beany back then; Jeff was shorter but also thin. So when I looked in the mirror I noticed that I was the only one with a little belly. "I'm fat!" I announced.

"You're not fat," my mother said, scurrying between rooms while getting ready. "You just ate. If you don't want to get fat, don't eat anything more tonight."

I stood there idly turning this way and that, examining my profile and deciding not to eat at church. As I look back upon that moment I realize that I was not fat. Not even overweight. I had a slightly different body style than my brothers, perhaps, but no one would have, or did, call me fat.

Something significant and private did happen in my world that night, however. It did not have to be a big deal, and I don't think I thought of it as such then, though it is significant that I still remember it: my resolve to not eat dissolved almost as soon as I saw the goodies. I say "almost" because I *started* with the proper commitment. I wasn't hungry. I felt full. And Mom had said, in passing, "If you don't want to get fat, don't eat any more tonight." Fair enough. But seeing everyone else enjoying my favorite stuff did me in.

This was not even a potluck dinner, which at the Oakwood Bible Church in those days featured world championship artery cloggers. Nobody cared much about fat percentages back then, and at a potluck at our church—and probably any other as well—you could load up on thousands of fatty, salty, greasy, sugary, tasty calories in a warm, loving, spiritual setting forever associated with happiness.

But on New Year's Eve we went to church after supper, so the banquet table of delights didn't have the usual casseroles, chicken, burgers, meatballs, meatloaf, and pasta. New Year's was a time for treats, so it was cake and pie and ice cream and brownies and cookies and fudge.

We were typically rambunctious kids, but Mom and Dad kept a fairly tight rein. We were not to load our plates with more than a couple of desserts—at least at one time. My brothers, and all the other normal-sized kids, overate at such functions, just as most adults did. But we had all learned to do it as politely as possible. (Not like a kid at a church I attended later who came back from the dessert table with nine squares of chocolate cake—looking as if he were about to serve his friends—and proceeded to eat them all. I may have found that disgusting and boorish, but he hadn't eaten any more than I had. I simply had mine one at a time and was more varied in my selection.)

During the New Year's Eve fun and games in 1956, however, I hadn't sat in the circle in the Fellowship Hall with a loaded paper plate on my lap and a cup of punch in my hand. I didn't make a big deal of it when people asked if I was going to have anything or why I wasn't. I didn't say I didn't want to get fat. I didn't have plans to eat secretly. It was only later, when we were horsing around during those hours between choruses and formal games and the midnight prayer, when I got a yen for something tasty.

The leftover desserts were on a main table, and people made occasional forays back for more. I was a brownie freak, but a couple of families had brought not just brownies, but brownies with frosting. Could there have been anything more delicious? The crunchy-edged, chewy, chocolatey cake of the brownie, made easier to chew and enjoy by that cool, smooth, buttery chocolate icing! I'm sorry to tell you, but when I see that famous little sign posted above scales all over the world that reads, "Nothing tastes as good as being thin feels," I think of those brownies and mutter, "Not!"

By the time I got back to my friends, my first brownie was gone and I wanted another. Over the course of the evening I gorged on those things as long as they lasted, one at a time. Had anyone kept track that night, they would have noticed that I had more brownies than anyone else, adult or child. In fact, I'm sure I consumed more brownie mass than anyone else consumed in total dessert mass. I had them one at a time; I don't recall even using a plate. I hadn't planned to eat, you'll recall.

It didn't seem monumental at the time. I knew I would probably "make myself sick," as adults always said. I didn't see this as the first step toward a lifetime of gluttony or obesity. It was simply a stupid, childish thing to do—something almost anyone can remember doing at one time or another, regardless of his current size and shape. I know people who've never had to worry about their weight who occasionally gorge and later groan about it.

But I do recall wandering to bed that night—the first time I had ever been allowed to stay up that late—and catching a tired-eyed glimpse of myself in the full-length mirror. That little distended belly was really pushing against my shirt, much more so than after supper. Mom had said not to eat more if I was worried about getting fat. I had eaten more than ever, and now I *was* fat.

In reality, of course, I wasn't. I was merely uncomfortable. I was so stuffed I had trouble sleeping. And I hadn't, as far as I know, triggered anything physically. Mentally I may have allowed myself to think I was now different from my brothers. I couldn't imagine their having done that, and they were certainly never going to be fat.

Photos from the year and a half or so after that show no hints of fatness on my part. I was still basically lean and athletic. I was beginning to love softball and swimming, and I recall being a fast runner, though I was still in the shadows of my older brothers athletically. Jim was long-legged and strong, and Jeff was already a budding sprinter. We were active, fun-loving, and close.

A couple of other vivid memories from that period are both of my dad. One is of him standing before that same mirror in his new police sergeant's dress uniform. I wasn't old enough to understand the significance, but it was clear that Dad was happy and Mom was proud. He eventually became a chief of police, but that promotion was the beginning of his rise.

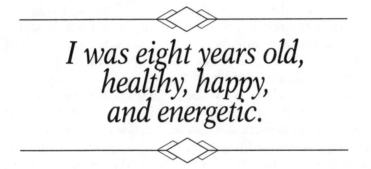

I was eight years old, healthy, happy, and energetic.

I also remember Dad playing softball with us. He pitched to us between our garage and the neighbor's, which was very close. Dad had to catch any line drives to keep them from breaking the neighbor's garage window. Jim was the only one of us who could hit the ball over the neighbor's garage, and that became my ambition in life. I was almost big enough by the following summer, but the closest I got was hitting a ball onto the roof and seeing it roll up and over. I couldn't believe the thrill, even though it didn't sky over like Jim's shots.

The next summer we moved a block away to a bigger house where we each had our own room. I recall announcing to my mother's parents: "Jim has his own room. Jeff has his own room. I have my own room. Mom and Dad still have to share a room, but that's only because we put the TV in the other bedroom."

The new place had a big driveway for basketball, a big backyard for running and playing catch, a perfect setup in front for playing Wiffle ball, and a scary, dark basement with a tunnel to the garage that legend said was built by gangsters during Prohibition.

We were still walking distance from the elementary and junior high schools and their playgrounds, the local swimming hole, and baseball diamonds. I was eight years old, healthy, happy, and energetic. It seemed I played every day from dawn till sundown.

That summer would blend into all the other summers of my childhood had it not been so fatefully eventful. Just after school was out I came down with the measles. If memory serves, my brother Jeff had them too. The family generally shared such maladies. I'll never forget when I was four and the three of us had our tonsils removed the same day and got our picture on the front page of the *Kalamazoo Gazette*. A year or so later we all had the chicken pox at once.

As soon as I was over the measles, I was back at all the summer's fun. Back then I had the idea that there was a year between school terms, when in reality there were about twelve weeks. Still, I wanted to pack in all the activity I could. Every day it was softball at the school diamond from just after breakfast till midafternoon when Mom took us to Oakwood Beach. In later years I would be embarrassed by my weight and either avoided swimming or carefully chose my spots. But in the summer of 1958, the lifeguard told my mother I swam like a fish. I was in the water for hours at a time and thought nothing of swimming to a raft halfway across the lake, resting, and swimming back.

But two weeks after getting over the measles, I got them again. That wasn't supposed to happen. No one in our orbit had heard of such a thing. Some said I had tried to become active again too quickly. Others said it was a different strain of the disease. I didn't know about such things, but that sounded logical. This bout hit me harder. The red spots were more severe, and I had more than the normal fever. I was wiped out, couldn't do anything, and felt bad that the summer's activities were delayed—not just for me but for Mom as well. She had to stay home with a sick kid, no fun for either of us.

After the spots went away and I should have been feeling better, I still felt logy and my joints were stiff, particularly my knees and ankles. I had to grab furniture as I walked, and I went upstairs on all fours. Then one morning I got up and could barely move. I tried to stand but fell to my knees. I'll never forget calling down to my father that I couldn't walk, couldn't even stand.

I had been one to exaggerate in the past. To my shame, I once faked a leg injury to get another kid to retrieve my sled and pull me on it. Somehow this time Dad knew it was no snow job. There was panic in my voice. And there's nothing an eight-year-old wants less than immobility when coming out of an illness.

I had to be carried down the stairs. I was scared, and from the looks on my parents' faces I could tell they were too.

4

The Metamorphosis

My measles had been treated symptomatically, and though our family doctor was intrigued by my having two bouts with the disease in the same month, he had not been as alarmed as everyone else.

Later that day my fever came roaring back with such intensity that I was delirious. I tried to stay under the covers in my parents' bed and "sweat it out," but occasionally I had to stick out a toe to cool off. At some point I must have crawled to the couch in the living room because that's where I found myself hours later, family members coming into and going out of focus. I might have enjoyed the attention, but this was big-league stuff for someone my age. I don't remember it, but my mother has told me that at one point I whispered, "Mom, I don't think I'm going to make it."

She called the doctor again. He asked to see me when I was up to it but said not to move me while in the throes of a high fever. He prescribed more aspirin, of course, and said to let him know if the fever didn't break in due time.

Ironically, once the fever broke, I felt wonderful. But my ankles still wouldn't support me, so the next morning I was carried to the car and helped into the doctor's office with a parent on either side. I was frustrated and embarrassed. I don't recall all the tests, but one was an electrocardiogram, and I was fascinated by the squiggly-lined readouts and the doctor's attempts to interpret them for me. The bottom line: a rheumatic condition, brought about by two separate cases of measles, overexertion, and an unusually high fever.

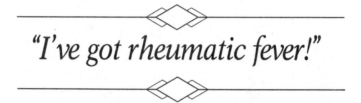

"I've got rheumatic fever!"

I didn't know what all that meant, but Mom—the wordsmith—tried to tell me. The doctor was worried that my heart had been damaged, and he wanted me in the hospital. I knew how serious it all was when, despite how normal and cheery I felt, I went directly from the doctor's office to Borgess Hospital. Mom told me I was the only one of her three boys to have been born there, so it would be like going where I belonged.

I was the strangest looking sick kid you ever saw. I was bright-eyed, talkative, smiling, loving every second of the attention. I talked to all the nurses and aides and doctors, eagerly opened my cards, loved visitors, and had a great time. As I was a Protestant in a Catholic hospital, Catholic clergy made no official visits, but when the occasional priest or nun caught a glimpse of me having such a good time, they would stop in and ask what in the world was wrong with me. By then my diagnosis had been upgraded (or I should say downgraded), and I would perkily announce, "I've got rheumatic fever!"

Once a priest said, "I'm not supposed to do this, but let me pray for you." I was struck by the fact that he didn't close his eyes, that he fingered his beads and cross as he prayed, and that he spoke in a foreign language.

My mother thanked him for his kindness, and when he left she asked, "Do you know what he was saying?" (She had studied Latin in high school and is a medical transcriptionist today.)

"Not really," I said. "Somethin' about wantin' to play dominoes with somebody!"

But not everything was fun and games. There were dark times. When there were no visitors or anything else to occupy my time, I dreaded my every-morning injection. I had learned that word quickly enough. No one could get away with talking about my shot by calling it an injection. I was onto them. And I learned to relax my rear end and not tighten up to take most of the sting away from the shot.

I also didn't understand how I could feel so good and still not be allowed out of bed, even to go to the bathroom. That was the height of indignity: bedpans! And being bathed in bed by a nurse or an aide! Once I was mortified when I was perched atop the bedpan, covered with a blanket, and an aide came in for my bath. My dad told her, "He's currently indisposed." She apologized and left, and I learned a couple of new words. She had to have wondered why I appeared so tall in the bed!

I was still young enough to not want to be left alone, but Mom and Dad were both working and had two other boys to take care of. Jim and Jeff could not visit me, but occasionally they waved from the grounds outside.

I always cried when Mom and Dad traded shifts sitting with me and then Dad had to get back to work in the early afternoon. He assured me they would be back in the evening and that there would be plenty of visitors, cards, and staff to keep me company during the daylight hours.

Every night they would come back to the hospital after dinner and sit with me until bedtime. The drink cart would come around, and I would order ginger ale. I don't remember why. To this day, when I have it occasionally, I am transported back to that time and place and the strange mixture of emotions: feeling great, having fun, dreading that shot, needing Mom or Dad there—and soon enough getting tired of it all.

One night when they were delayed, the drink cart lady came and asked what I wanted. She assumed it would be my usual, but I wanted a change. Chocolate milk? Cola? I couldn't decide. I thought and thought and simply couldn't make a decision. I was touched by her patience as she suggested everything from orange juice to milk. But I took my thirty-plus pills a day—mainly penicillin, aspirin, sulfa, and cortisone—with orange juice, so that didn't appeal.

When she had been through the list twice, she suggested that maybe I didn't want anything to drink just then. I couldn't imagine ever passing up a treat, but she was right. I nodded, melancholy, missing Mom and Dad, relieved to have made a decision by choosing nothing. Thirty-five years later that insignificant little incident is lodged in my brain.

When it was time for me to go to sleep, Mom and Dad would pray with me, help me memorize John chapter 3, and turn out the lights. Then they would play Scrabble by a sliver of light from the bathroom until I fell asleep. If they made any attempt to leave before I was out, I'd tell them, and they'd wait. I weep to this day remembering that sensitivity. I was not demanding, and they never accused me of such. They simply knew how hard this had to be on a little boy, and they made it as easy for me as possible.

Pictures from that period show battle-weary parents and a beaming kid confined to the bed in which they should have been resting. Mom has dark circles under her eyes, and the strain shows on my dad's face. He was thirty-five and she thirty-two, and I didn't have a clue as to what they were going through.

In spite of how wonderful I felt, I didn't know until years later that my tests were not coming back as positively as the doctor had hoped. Every day I felt better and assumed that it wouldn't be long before I was back on the ball diamond. But a week stretched to two and then to almost three before I was allowed to go home, still bedridden for yet another several months.

Years and years later I was teaching a writers conference when I met an editor from *Guideposts* magazine who asked me if I was aware that my mother had entered the annual writers' contest. I was not. "Her story is not going to win," she told me, "but if she doesn't show it to you, ask to see it."

And so eventually I did. She had hoped to win, of course, and planned for the publication of the story to be a surprise to me. It was about my brief period in the hospital as an eight-year-old, and, although I had heard much of the story before, Mom's story finally drove home a parent's perspective. She told of those first few days, when I was so merry that people wondered what I was doing in a hospital bed. She knew the awful truth that not only did I belong there, but also my blood test results were discouraging. No one told me, of course, but there was the possibility that I might never come home.

Mom told of praying, of telling God, "You can't take my child. Please don't." Only when she realized that I was not hers but His and that He could do whatever He wished did she break down and release me to His will. Her story recounts that tearful letting go, and how I almost immediately began to improve. It has been only in adulthood, as a father, that I have understood the deep feelings of ownership, love, and protectiveness a parent has for a child.

That was such a brief patch on the embroidery of my life, and yet distinct memories remain. My Sunday school teacher sneaked in a chocolate shake for me. A boy down the hall wandered in with a rubber dart gun, and we took turns sticking the darts to the ceiling, waiting for them to drop. (A nurse finally chased him off, telling him that I wasn't up to that much activity yet.)

I got cards every day, including a series that continued for a week, each succeeding card answering a silly question from the previous. I got a haircut, and clippings fell in my Silly Putty, which also turned dark as I used it to offset print from the comics.

I had my picture taken with my favorite nurse. Several doctors loved my fake hypodermic syringe, which had a spring-loaded "needle" that retracted when it came in contact with the skin and appeared to be drawing blood. One first-year resident from India brought someone in almost every day to watch him *give* blood at the hands of a young patient.

I even got my first taste of women's rights way back then. Most of the nurse's aides—all female—said they were studying to become nurses. But one said that she wanted to be a doctor. "I didn't know girls could be doctors," I said.

"You learn something new every day," she said.

After two weeks and five days in room 518, I was allowed to go home. I was stunned at what I had forgotten about the rest of the hospital since I had been wheeled in. It didn't look at all like what I had imagined from the sounds coming from up and down the hall. The elevator was tiny, manually operated, and noisy. I got a glimpse of the little girl across the hall who was confined to a Stryker Frame and whose whimpering I heard every day. Whenever I complained of being bedridden, I was reminded of her. She could not move.

The wheelchair ride to our car made me dizzy, and I felt embarrassed to be in my pajamas during the day. I didn't think to ask whether I would still have to use bedpans at home and was greatly disappointed to find out that I did. The TV had been moved out of that extra bedroom on the first floor, and that became my new spot, day and night.

I still enjoyed being the center of attention, but I was getting tired of that bed. My focus became when I could get up, at least to go to the bathroom, and whether I would be walking in time for school in the fall. I was going into fourth grade and would turn nine that first month of school. I couldn't wait.

I also looked forward to getting back to church. In Sunday school, I came to painfully realize, I had been an obnoxious, big mouth, know-it-all. In junior church I had been named Junior Pastor, which didn't involve much but which I interpreted as some sort of a spiritual accomplishment. I now realize that the leader wanted somebody who knew lots of Bible verses and could read.

September came and went and I was still in bed. I had a tutor. The doctor visited weekly and often brought an injection. By then I was so grateful that I didn't have a daily shot that I was proud to just roll over and take it. I also became adept at taking my weekly bloodletting (for tests) without wincing.

The doctor began to prepare me for the pain and awkwardness of walking again for the first time. He said I would need help but that he would like me to take it slowly and not resort to crutches or a cane. My knees and ankles would be weak, my muscles atrophied. I was a bigger boy, he said, than when I first fell ill, because I had been inactive.

That was something I had not thought of and didn't really know. As far as I know, there are no pictures of me in bed at home, so all I recall from that period are the ones of a happily smiling kid in the hospital with friends, family, and medical staff. I didn't see the change that was happening to my body.

One advantage of being at home was that occasionally Mom or Dad would carry me to the screened-in front porch for a brief change of scenery. I noticed after a while that Mom struggled more to lift me and finally had to leave such things to Dad. That should have been a clue.

But despite all the talk of taking my first steps, no one had given me permission. I just waited and waited. Finally, one day when no one was in the room, I slid my foot down the side of the bed to the floor and put my weight on it. It felt strange, the ankle tender, but I was encouraged. I sensed I could do this. I quickly returned to bed. Then I felt guilty. Had I done something I wasn't supposed to do? I was a kid with a fragile conscience, often feeling the need to confess, and so I did. I told my mother what I had done. She smiled. "That's what the doctor has been waiting for," she said. "He said you would let us know when you were ready to try walking."

She called and told him what I had done, and he gave permission for me to be helped from my room, through the living room, to the bathroom. Mom and Dad stayed close, but I wanted to do it myself. I swung my legs over the side of the bed and stood, feeling the blood rush from my head. I steadied myself and took a couple of steps to where I could support myself by the door frame. Then, with Mom and Dad close and encouraging me to take it slowly, I carefully managed to work my way through the big house to the bathroom.

It was there alone, standing at the sink to get my own drink of water, that I got the shock of my life. I didn't recognize the little boy in the mirror, because there was none. I had weighed sixty-nine pounds at the doctor's office at the beginning of the summer. Now, in November, a few weeks from reentering my school and church worlds, I had ballooned. Staring back at me from that mirror was a pale, moon-faced kid whose smile had faded.

Mom asked from the other side of the door if I was all right. I told her I would be right out, and I stepped on the scales. In five short months I had gained more than fifty pounds. I was nine years old and weighed 125 pounds. I was no longer an energetic child. I wasn't the sick kid about to come back to school.

I was just plain fat.

5

Facing the World Again

I said nothing to anyone about my shock over my new body. What could be said? It wasn't their fault. I don't recall having overeaten during that time, but we didn't know what we do today about fat and cholesterol. I had plenty of eggs and beef and sweets and whole milk.

The doctor told me that one of the new types of cortisone I had been given might make my hair thin on top but might make me grow a moustache. We all thought that pretty funny. I decided I wanted a handlebar moustache, but nothing ever appeared on my upper lip until it was supposed to several years later. My hair has been thin ever since, and I even had the beginnings of a bald spot before age ten, but it never bothered me.

The doctor also told me that the medication may have affected my metabolism. He explained that metabolism was the process by which my body produced tissue and energy and waste from food and air and water. I didn't understand much, but I came away with the idea that I might have to eat less than the normal person or exercise more to keep from gaining more weight and certainly to lose any.

I need to say, however, that in light of what we have learned about cortisone and metabolism, and given what I have learned about my body through various weight loss and control efforts, I have become convinced that my doctor was wrong. After a lifetime of obsession with weight, fat, food, diet, body, and all things related, I can look back on what happened to and with me with much clearer lenses.

This will come as no surprise to you, but what happened to me is the same as would happen to anyone else in a similar circumstance. Regardless of the weight control program someone is on, if he consumes more calories than he burns, he gains weight. If he consumes fewer than he burns, he loses weight. Yes, some people have higher metabolic rates than others, men over women, for instance. And yes, certain medicines and physical conditions can affect metabolism. The body itself will change its metabolic rate if it senses it is being starved. (I wish it would do the opposite too and kick into high gear when it feels it is being overfed, but, no, it simply stores the excess as fat.)

I went from being a typical Tasmanian devil of an eight-year-old to a sedentary, inactive, bedridden kid who still had a big appetite.

Anyway, despite using my "ruined metabolism from medication taken as a child" as a lifelong excuse for my weight problem, it doesn't hold water. Every time I have gotten serious about weight loss and have consumed fewer calories than I burned, I lost quickly. My metabolism is fine. It's normal to above-normal for a male, and I have proven that I can average as high as a five-pound-per-week loss for months.

What happened to me was that I went from being a typical Tasmanian devil of an eight-year-old to a sedentary, inactive, bedridden kid who still had a big appetite. I suppose a very careful diet could have made a difference, but who was going to deprive a sick kid of one of the great joys of life?

My first foray into public came late that fall when I went back to Sunday school and junior church. It might have been easier if kids had stared or even made fun of me. That would come later, but my perception and recollection is that they were so astounded at my appearance that they didn't know how to react. I don't know if I expected a welcome-back banner and a party or everyone gathering around to see how I was or what. I do know they had been prepared for my return. They had been kept up to date on my progress and had been praying for me.

When I entered the room of about fifty kids, everyone turned and looked. The leader said, "Welcome back, Jerry," and everyone looked away again. Right or wrong, what I read in their looks was, "Good grief, what happened to him?" I have seen a picture of me with my brothers, taken in the backyard that afternoon. We're all dressed up, of course. I'm smiling, but I can see the pain in my eyes. I look twice the size of my brothers, and that huge, round face makes me look older.

At school I had enjoyed the "smartest kid in the class" tag since kindergarten. But, now, going into fourth grade a couple of months late, I was behind. With my tutor I had been on a different pace, but that wasn't the worst of it. I would quickly get back into the swing of things academically. What was worse was that I had been the organizer. We had softball teams, dodge ball games, all kinds of stuff. I was always in the middle of it—before school, during recess, over the lunch hour, and after school.

But now I was out of the mix. I had to take it easy, sit out from gym class for a while, not roughhouse and run. My new teacher was sensitive and nice. She had taught my big brother a few years before and had fond memories of what a good student and voracious reader he was.

But for some reason there was no desk for me for my first couple of weeks back. So, in addition to feeling alien to my old friends and politely ignored by them because of my new appearance, I had to sit at a table away from the rows of desks too. It was too wide to fit into the layout of the room, which was exactly how *I* felt.

I poured myself into catching up academically, and much as my mother tried to get me to slow down physically, it wasn't long before I was back to my old, energetic ways. I didn't have the endurance I once had, and though I could play all day, I couldn't run long distances without shortness of breath, which is true even today.

Before long I got a normal desk, worked my way back into the fun stuff, and became one of the guys again. I was, however, the fat kid, and no amount of athletic ability or academic prowess changed that. I don't recall how I ate in those days, but I do know I gained thirty pounds over the next two years. So, though I was more active, I was also consuming a lot more food.

I had been praying for a baby brother or sister for a couple of years, and when I was ten, in fifth grade, little brother Jay came along. I was thrilled. Perhaps his becoming the center of attention affected me, however. I wasn't aware of it, but I may have resorted to food to fill a void.

One night while Mom was still in the hospital recovering from the delivery and we boys were staying with friends, we all went to a roller skating party. Having a few dollars in my pocket and no parent to control me, I gorged on snacks at the rink. By the end of the evening I was stuffed to the gills, but I realized I had enough money left for a butterscotch shake. That sounded terribly intriguing, so I bought one.

On my way out to the car with the others, I tripped in the darkness over a carstop in the parking lot and was heading for the asphalt before I knew it. Yet somehow I managed to hit the deck without dropping or even spilling that shake. That's how important it was to me.

You'd think there's always room in a full tummy for a little more liquid, but I think I hit a new personal record for fullness that evening. I fully expected to be sick in the night, but I just waited it out and felt fine by morning. Was I missing my parents? Tense over the new baby brother I had not yet seen?

Aware that my life was about to change? Or simply overreacting to a little freedom?

Who can say? I had developed, however, even at that young age, a prodigious appetite and the ability to more than fulfill it.

Growing taller as I approached puberty should have made my weight look more normal for my frame. But I continued to gain, which simply made me a taller, bigger version of the fat, nine-year-old fourth grader who emerged from his sick bed.

I cringed to see composite class pictures, where our individual head shots were pasted together on one sheet. There were all the lean, defined cheekbones of Mr. Knuth's sixth grade class at Oakwood Elementary School, along with one double-chinned fat face of a boy who looked older than his years.

I have to say that my most painful memory as a fat child came in the sixth grade when it was time for our annual physical fitness tests. I didn't do so well in the 600-yard run, but then few did besides the exceptional athletes. I did surprisingly well in the sprints, won the softball throw, and placed high in the shuttle run and the standing long jump. I enjoyed surprising people with my speed and mobility.

But then came the day when we were measured and weighed. Our coach, a sensitive Christian and a former local star athlete, had each of us step on the scale, then he softly announced our weights to one of the girls in our class, who recorded them. The coach used one of those upright physician's scales, where the heavy weight is set at fifty-pound increments and the smaller weight is slid along another bar pound by pound. Most of the kids in the class, of course, could be weighed with the big weight at fifty and the smaller weight adding another forty or so pounds. I remember one of the pretty girls weighing in the high eighties and squealing, "Oh, I've gained!" I hated her.

Needless to say, I dreaded being weighed and having anyone know how much. I was gratified to notice, however, that the rest of the class quickly lost interest in the process and idly chatted as they waited their turns. When my name was called, however, the room fell deadly silent. I stepped on the scale and turned my head away as the coach slid the big weight from the fifty to the hundred mark, then started sliding the smaller weight.

When the balance had not budged even after he had added forty-nine pounds, he moved the big weight to 150 and slid the small one back to zero. Then he turned to the girl with the clipboard, known for her big mouth, and gave her a look both she and I interpreted as "Keep your mouth shut."

I'll always be grateful for his attempt to protect me. As quietly as he could, he simply said, "One-five-six," and with that the class erupted.

"A hundred and fifty-six!"

"Wow! Did you hear that?"

"Oh, man! My dad doesn't weigh that much!"

Amid the continuing tumult, the coach bellowed, "Hold it down!" Again I was grateful that he didn't start a lecture about being kind. I simply smiled and shook my head as if I was as surprised and amused as everyone else.

6

Sticks and Stones May Break My Bones, but Words Will Break My Heart

Once I tripped trotting up some stairs and missed a step. No problem, except that a relative said, "Nice play, ox." It was something everybody said back then—a joke, a teasing insult. Someone might have just as naturally said it to one of my lean brothers, and they probably did. But it cut me deeply.

Another time an adult was lecturing one of my friends as I stood alongside. At the end of the conversation he pointed to me and said, "That goes for you too, fatso."

Friends of my mother told their toddlers in front of me, "You be good now, or Jerry will sit on you."

One of the great joys of my life, after having been a life-long softball addict, was to see Little League baseball come to town. I threw myself into it from age ten. When I was eleven I made the Oakwood all-star team that surprised everybody in its first year of tournament competition by finishing fourth in the state. Some of the greatest memories of my life came from that period, and my goal was to became a major league baseball player.

The next year I was one of six returning twelve-year-olds, and we won the state championship. We missed going to Williamsport, Pennsylvania, for the Little League World Series by one game, and the team that beat us wound up finishing second in the world. Pictures back then show me a happy, smiling kid doing what he loved best, but there is one photo that's painful.

The local paper ran a shot of us six returnees, and it just happened that the other five were either exactly average for their ages or much smaller. I am at one end of the line with my specially made uniform, nearly twice the size of the others.

Sometimes, inexplicably, I brought such humiliation on myself. One night my mother, the choir director, had the choir over for a party. Our house was full of people. When the time came for refreshments, Mom laid out several pieces of pie on the dining room table. Choir members stood in line, and my dad prayed. I had my eye on the one double-sized portion, so as soon as I heard the "amen" I grabbed it.

Mom immediately chastised me and made me put it back. I was humiliated, and rightly so. It was a boorish, typically self-centered, childish thing to do, and she was more concerned with my impoliteness than that I was a fat kid wanting a big piece of pie. The irony of it was that everyone saw and heard, so no one had the heart to take that piece. When it was all that was left, I got it anyway.

With the onset of puberty came other confusing complications. I didn't like the idea of growing up and becoming a man. Maybe that was because I already looked like one, while inside I felt like the child that I was. All the attendant body changes seemed distasteful to me, and it took me a long time to get used to the idea that my childhood was history.

By now I was aware of a huge appetite, but it was not unlike my brothers and my peers. As we developed musculature and were awash in new hormones, we ate. I was as active as ever, fully involved in sports, and I was getting a lot taller. By eighth grade I was about 5'9", and I excelled in physical education.

We lifted weights. We ran. I actually got my 600-yard run down to a respectable time for a big kid. I have to admit, my weight started looking better on me. My face had more definition, and as my upper body developed, my waist didn't look so big. I was still gaining weight, however, and even though much of it was new muscle, I was still self-conscious about how big I was.

I remember standing in line to be weighed in eighth-grade gym class and actually rocking on my toes, almost imperceptibly, hoping to make myself sweat off a pound or two before I reached the scales. Two years after that humiliating sixth-grade weigh-in, I was up twenty-four pounds to 180. Strangely, however, this was less humiliating. Kids came right out and asked me what I weighed, and they seemed impressed. Maybe I didn't look so fat, but just big. Even the coach exulted that I was the size of a man. I felt better about myself.

The spring of my eighth-grade year, 1963, my dad became chief of police in Elk Grove Village, Illinois, a northwestern suburb of Chicago. At the end of the school year, the family would join him there. Frankly, I couldn't wait. All those stories you hear about kids not wanting to leave their churches, schools, friends, homes, and all that—that wasn't me. I was one who always liked new things, turning over a new leaf, starting over, resolving to do better.

I left Michigan like a bad habit, though I really had no reason to. I had many friends, many wonderful memories, and frequently have found myself returning nostalgically over the years. But for some reason I was ready for a change.

By the time I was a high school senior I was a shade over six feet tall and weighed in the low 230s.

Though Dad made more money, our brand-new but smaller home cost so much more than the one in Oakwood that we were no better off financially. My older brothers and I all went to a beautiful, new, huge public high school. Jim and I went out for football, Jeff for cross country. Jim made the varsity. Jeff made the frosh-soph team. Because I was big and strong, already up another couple of inches and thirty pounds—to 210 —everybody assumed I should be a football player. That was why I went out, but that didn't make me a player. I endured a couple of weeks of excruciating two-a-day football practices before breaking my arm. I was so thrilled to be through with football I'd have probably broken my arm earlier if I had thought of it. All I cared about was baseball. Football, though I always loved watching it, had been a bad idea for me.

Baseball was still my game. I stayed close to the athletes by being an equipment manager with the basketball team while my arm was healing, biding my time till spring. I made the freshman A team as starting first baseman batting fifth, but in the second game a runner came down on my leg on a close play and I suffered ligament damage to my knee. Nowadays arthroscopic surgery would probably have had me back in action within a year, but in those days radical knee surgery was the only option and there was little hope of ever returning to form.

I gave up my dream, opted against surgery, and turned to sportswriting to stay close to the sports scene. I almost immediately realized that I had found my niche, and I've never looked back. Sure, I would rather have been a big league baseball star, but I have come to learn that even if I had become the best high school player in Illinois—which I was not—the odds would have been heavy against my making the pros. Even at the point where a superstar is drafted out of college, his chances of making a living in the majors are 1 in 100.

I loved writing and covering sports, and though I stayed active in church softball, intramurals, and pickup games, I was getting my regular exercise only in gym class and found myself gaining weight again. By the time I was a high school senior I was a shade over six feet tall and weighed in the low 230s. Pictures from that period show that I learned to carry my weight well. Few would have guessed me at over 200 pounds, but I still got the occasional cut in the locker room: "Jenkins, when are you gonna do something about that gut?"

I had also begun dating, and my girlfriend was not sympathetic about my weight. I worked hard at eating less and working out more because I didn't want her to be embarrassed, but of course that was the wrong motivation. I was desperately seeking unconditional love, whether I knew it or not, and when she once referred to my weight as "disgusting," I sensed the beginning of the end. It would not have worked for many reasons, but the breakup a couple of years later was still traumatic.

The summer between high school and college also saw me gain thirty pounds. I played church softball once a week, which was not enough to make up for increased consumption. I'm sure I was worried about leaving home and a new phase of life, but I was not aware of stress then and have only recently surrendered to the possibility that my compulsive overeating is even somewhat triggered by outside sources.

I became convinced that I was just a big eater who loved food and was undisciplined. What triggered my overeating? Had you suggested stress, tension, disappointment, unhappiness, I would have denied it. I never needed a reason, so if I was eating to mask some deep inner need, I was doing a good job of it. I was unaware of any eating triggers other than the sun coming up every morning.

Happy? Eat.

Sad? Eat.

Uptight? Eat.

Celebrating? Eat.

7

The Parallel Path

You could easily look at the foregoing and see a neurotic, unhappy, overly sensitive fat kid with a low self-image. What a sad, depressing way to grow up, you might think.

On the contrary. If you are a fellow struggler, you'll recognize that the story I have told so far is the private one. These were things I never talked about to anyone. Occasionally my mother would encourage or warn me in some area related to my weight, assuring me that she merely wanted to protect me from a lifetime of fat-related pain. She always said these things sympathetically and lovingly, so I was not wounded by insensitivity.

But otherwise, outwardly, I was a happy kid. And before I get back to the chronological story of my gradual but steady weight gain, let me clarify that I did not let my problem affect me inwardly much either. I doubt I thought more about my eating habits than anyone else did about theirs. Everybody binged occasionally. But I decided I couldn't get away with it because of this metabolism malady caused by the medication during my childhood illness.

Generally I look back on a largely happy childhood and adolescence. As a youngster I was fun-loving and enjoyed other kids. I loved school and Sunday school, and though I now realize that I was a typically obnoxious third child, trying to control or even dominate my environment when outside the hierarchy of my own family (where I was low man on the totem pole), I still have fond memories.

I excelled in sports and most school subjects. I was selected one of only about twenty sixth graders in Kalamazoo to attend a special summer school for gifted students. I was a spelling champion and already enjoyed writing stories, though I never dreamed of becoming a writer.

Teachers had to deal with my tendency to interrupt without raising my hand, to comment on everything, or to make a joke. Ironically, even with my love of talking (I realize now it was from a need for attention, of course), I was petrified of speaking publicly. In eighth grade I prayed earnestly every day that I would not be the one called upon to do his oral book report. I died a thousand deaths, only to find day by day that my prayer had been answered. It was always someone else.

Each day I came prepared, yet dreading the inevitable. I lived in turmoil for more than a month while one by one my classmates were called to the front of the room for their presentations. Finally, when everyone else had done theirs, the teacher said, "Have I missed anyone?"

I sat there silently, unable to believe my luck. Did God really care about such things? Then the teacher said, "Why, Mr. Jenkins, we haven't heard from you!" Had I gone first, rather than last, I'd have lived in comfort during all the other speeches!

Though I was somewhat of a wallflower in junior high, painfully progressing through the onset of puberty, in high school (in a new state) I seemed to blossom again. As a freshman I became such an incessant talker that people would often say so. I recall asking a friend if I had told him a certain story before. "Only about a thousand times," he said, walking away.

Waiting for the school bus home one day I was holding court with a bunch of kids, totally unaware that I was dominating the conversation until my brother said, "Why don't you just be quiet for a while?" That hurt. But we all need those midcourse adjustments occasionally.

As a sophomore in high school I was class clown, yet when called upon to address the class I was nearly catatonic. My mouth was dry, my hands shook, I was short of breath. My speeches were the shortest on record, and I found that if I resorted to humor and could gain a laugh or two, it was somehow easier. I was always graded down due to brevity, however.

When I started dating I gained a little more confidence. I became president of our high school Youth For Christ club and often regaled friends with from-memory renditions of comedian George Carlin's famous newscasts and commercials. Then my YFC director asked me to do the same for a big club meeting with groups from other schools. Why I agreed, I'll never know. He must have sensed my hesitancy, though I could not turn him down in front of my peers. He assured me that he would use a spotlight and that I would never see the faces of the crowd.

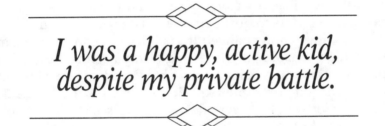

I was a happy, active kid, despite my private battle.

I recalled having made announcements over the school loud speaker occasionally and that I didn't suffer from stage fright because I couldn't see the people I was addressing. For my newscast I would sit at a table with a blanket draped over it so that it would look like a news desk and would hide my knocking knees. I would also wear a hat—why I don't know, because TV news people never did. It was just a prop to make me look like an old-fashioned reporter, but it also hid me.

And the spotlight did the trick. I could see no one, but I could hear the laughter. What a tonic! After dying with dread all day, I was a hit! The discomfort was worth the response after all! I began doing that little comedy routine all over the place, and it was a real confidence booster.

I was no big man on campus at our huge school (more than 2,000 students), but I did become sports editor of the school paper. Eventually I had articles published in the *Chicago Tribune* and *Campus Life* magazine, which would help propel me into journalism.

So I was a happy, active kid, despite my private battle. In fact, because of my body style, few people were aware how heavy I was. I was big enough to be the brunt of jokes, but in clothes I might have appeared more solid than I was. I could have just as easily looked like a body builder as a fat guy, because through high school my chest was bigger than my stomach. As few people as possible saw me without a shirt.

Another parallel life at this time was spiritual. Having been raised in a Christ-honoring, godly family and becoming a believer at a young age, I was comfortable and happy in church. As a young teen at camp I was shaken by a message from a slightly older friend of mine, John Ankerberg, who challenged us to "live for Christ by God's grace even if you have to stand alone." He urged us to quit being secret-service Christians.

I was moved and changed that night. I began carrying my Bible to high school and witnessing to my friends. Several became Christians and joined our YFC Campus Life club. My brother Jeff had the same experience, and during his senior and my junior years we were devout witnesses at our school. I was the only kid in my school to go to Moody Bible Institute, and, rather than be embarrassed by that, I was proud of it. It gave many opportunities for me to tell people what Moody was all about, and that led to more witnessing opportunities.

As a college freshman my weight fluctuated from about 260 to the low 240s when I was briefly ill, then up to about 275 by the end of the school year. Because I was now eighteen and my frame was maturing, my weight didn't show so much in my face. In fact, photos from that time make me appear large but not fat, and my face is fairly well-defined. From a photo you might guess me at about 200 pounds. I also learned how to dress, buying shirts larger than I needed and wearing my belt at the waist, not tucked under my stomach. It's amazing how some people fifty pounds lighter can look that much heavier because of how they wear their clothes and carry themselves.

People who saw me in person guessed me as high as 220–225, but never the fifty pounds heavier that I was. That cut both ways, of course. I knew the terrible truth that I was off the charts and unhealthy, yet, if people thought I looked OK, what was the difference?

It was during my year as a student at Moody that I became aware of the power of presence. I'm not sure I accepted the premise, but I certainly began to think about it. Though I didn't look as heavy as I was, still I was almost a hundred pounds heavier than the average freshman. Once guys got to know me and we became friends, they became more honest with me and told me what they had initially thought of me.

They had been intimidated, they said. I was a fast talker, a guy with ideas. When we all wanted to do something, they tended to defer to my ideas. This reaction was so common that I couldn't deny it, but I was totally—and I mean totally—unaware of it until it was occasionally pointed out to me.

Whatever power of personality I had was not intentional and was, in fact, the opposite of what I felt inside. My private turmoil over continuing to gain weight made me feel undisciplined. And the way I handled my new freedom, being away from home for the first time, proved I was indeed undisciplined. I managed my time poorly, had bad sleeping habits, ate all the meals that were provided, plus candy and ice cream junk from machines, and burgers at the local greasy spoons.

Often I would say, "I'll buy if you'll fly," meaning, "Go get us some burgers, and I'll pay for it." I wasn't a wealthy person. I had as little money as the next guy. But I began to see why I seemed intimidating or cocky or even pushy. As I say, I didn't feel it inside. In fact, I felt less than adequate because my life was not in control. Somehow, my size accentuated any false bravado or eagerness to be aggressive, so people were put off until they got to know me. Many mentioned that they had been, in essence, happy to oblige my wishes. Somebody had to make decisions for the group, they said, so why shouldn't it be a fun-loving guy like me who often offered to finance whatever the excursion?

When we talked frankly, sometimes even years hence, friends from that period admitted that my size must have had a lot to do with my impact. There is something parental or authoritative about being the largest person in the room. To me it was an embarrassment, but somehow it accentuated any emotion. If I was serious, I looked more serious. If I was upset, it was hard to mask. If I disagreed mildly, I seemed contentious. When having fun, I *really* appeared to have fun. Someone described me as a person with big appetites, not just for food, but for life, adventure, discussion, sports, you name it.

As you will see in chapter 17, I was otherwise unaware of the power of my presence due to my size until I lost my weight as a middle-aged adult. Having not realized its impact and import and having never consciously "used" it for effect, I never knew how subconsciously it affected my whole being—and it had been noticed as early as that freshman year at Moody.

You can see that my weight and my eating habits, though painful burdens, did not dominate my life at that time—at least not until I decided to let people in on my private battle. While playing church softball during the summer after my year at Moody I felt less mobile and my weight showed more in our uniforms. So I was intrigued when I heard a friend and his wife talk about the weight they had lost on a low-carbohydrate diet.

I asked a lot of questions and read a few sheets about it. What interested me was learning that many foods I enjoyed most were low in carbohydrates. I could eat all the beef I wanted, have a salad with mayonnaise, and lose pounds. This would mark the first time I had done anything seriously and systematically about my weight.

I was young and athletic, and my metabolism—though I didn't know it—was effective. The diet worked like a charm. I was staying away from breads and fruits, because of the weight-producing carbohydrates (which I couldn't have defined to save my life).

My rapid weight loss quickly became evident. I probably dropped twenty pounds and enjoyed the accolades of my friends and my girlfriend. I did not enjoy it, however, when everyone seemed to take an interest in what I ate or didn't eat. "I didn't know you could have that," they would say.

"Is that on your diet?"

"Are you off your diet?"

"Have you gained any weight back?"

When the scale showed I had gained back only three pounds, no one believed it. Rightly so, because when you're gaining, you look bigger and less comfortable even than when you've settled in to a new, higher weight.

I enjoyed the attention when I was losing, but I resented it when I was not. How people reacted to my diet or lack thereof became a silent gauge to me of whether they truly loved me. I wanted unconditional acceptance, and, though not assertive enough to say so at the time, I categorized people by how they responded to me.

Of course, the low-carbohydrate diet was unbalanced, led to cravings, was high in fat, and was doomed to failure. Had I stayed on it, I would have continued to lose or been able to maintain, because I was consuming fewer calories than I burned. But that amazing secret ("Just limit carbohydrate intake") was no panacea.

I continued to "watch" what I ate, especially in public. No one could understand my weight problems, because I seemed to eat no more than they did.

The next year, when my engagement ended after a long relationship and I began going to a local community college part time while pursuing my career as sports editor of a daily newspaper, I settled into a nearly suicidal lifestyle without knowing it and without realizing why.

I became almost totally sedentary. I was living at home, sleeping till noon. I went to school in the afternoon, got to the office three or four hours later, covered local high school sports in the evening, wrote my stories, developed my pictures, laid out my pages, and headed home near dawn.

The only exercise I got was working my way out of my small car and climbing into press boxes or prowling sidelines. I loved my job and seemed to do it well, but I was one troubled, unsettled person. No doubt the broken love relationship had a deeper effect on me than I was aware of, because the way I ate proved I was trying to fill some void. I was pursuing the career I wanted and had good friends. But my eating was out of control, and I didn't even think about exercise.

8

The Ugly Side

I warn you—this is one of the darker sides of my story. Not as dark as when I get to my conclusions about why I am a compulsive overeater, but ugly nonetheless. If you are a fellow struggler, you will painfully identify with it. If you are a civilian, you will not likely understand. I'm not sure I understand it myself, and certainly there is little to be gained in the way of a sense of well-being by revealing this much. I make myself vulnerable because it is the only way I know to tell the whole, truthful story and try to come to some conclusions.

The bare facts are that from the time I left Moody in the spring of 1968 and endured the breakup of a romance that had begun in high school, I began a meteoric increase in calorie consumption that had its natural result. I gained weight so quickly I could hardly stay in the same clothes for more than a couple of months at a time.

If you've endured such a period, you know the pain and the desperation. I didn't know what I wanted or what I was looking for. I was not aware of trying to fill a void or numb some pain, but doubtless that was all there. I told myself I loved food and enjoyed eating—which is also true.

I had a steady income, and my expenses consisted of only a car payment and a small stipend to my parents for living at home. I ate out most of the time, and I enjoyed anything and everything I wanted. My recollection of that period is that I ate almost constantly—much of the time, but not exclusively, alone.

Certainly not because I'm proud of it, but only to show how dangerous and destructive such a lifestyle can be I am going to make use of modern technology to try to get a bead on an average twenty-four-hour's caloric and fat intake. Today I keep track of everything I eat by computer, with a program from Parson's Technology called The Diet Analyst. It carries the nutritional content, calories, and fats of almost any food you can think of, including fast foods and brand-name products. Anything that is not already in its database can be plugged in with a few keystrokes. Here I will use its figures to show what I was doing to my body before age twenty-one, as I sped past 300 pounds for the first time.

As is typical for an out-of-control eater, I skipped breakfast. There are many theories about this. One is that the fat person eats so much close to bedtime that he cannot be hungry when he wakes up. Subconsciously he may also be telling himself that he will enjoy his lunch more if he has some semblance of hunger. In reality, he is consuming such mass quantities that he never allows himself real hunger. His body gets so used to constant fuel and excess resources that when his digestive process has started and his stomach is less than full, he thinks he's hungry.

We now know, of course, that even a huge overeater would do better to have something for breakfast, even if it increased his total caloric intake for the day, because it gets the digestive system going and tells the body it is being fed and does not have to go into a starvation-protecting mode.

Nonetheless, my typical day began late in the morning when I rose and skipped breakfast. Ironically, even though I was consuming mass quantities of food every day, it's likely that by lunchtime my body had decided to store as much fat as possible to counteract the "fast" that seemed to have begun when I went to bed and continued until I rolled into McDonald's on the way to community college.

There I would start my day with a minimum of two large sandwiches; back then they would have been double cheeseburgers, approximately equivalent to the Quarter-Pounder with

Cheese today. I would also have two orders of fries, a hot apple pie, a large Coke, and a chocolate shake.

Does anyone need that much lunch? Of course not. Few need that much in an entire day. Can anyone enjoy all that food? I did. Did the last bite taste as good as the first? Not entirely, but I ate quickly enough to stay ahead of my satiety mechanism (which tells the brain that the stomach has had enough), so I wasn't uncomfortable until about twenty minutes later when I wedged into my desk at school.

So, how had my day started? The double cheeseburgers would have been about 483 calories apiece, or 966. Of that total, 486 calories would have come from fat, or more than 50 percent. The two orders of fries totaled 640 calories, of which 48 percent came from fat. Back then the shakes were not low-fat as they are today, so the chocolate shake was 356 calories, of which 20 percent came from fat. The hot apple pie would have been 260 calories and more than 50 percent fat. A large Coke would have been 324 calories, mostly sugar.

So that first meal of the day would have totaled more than 2500 calories, 990 of those from fat, or 39 percent of the total.

Now let me be agonizingly clear. Even though that equals approximately the total whole day calorie intake of my present lifestyle (with fat percentages in the low 20s), I was just barely getting started. You're going to find my daily totals back then as astounding as I have, now that I have put the computer to work on them.

That beginning was only that, for I ate like that again at least twice, and often three times, in a twenty-four hour period, with snacks in between. If anything was offered at school—donuts, candy bars, chips, nuts—I accepted and probably had more than most. Discreetly, of course. You learn to nibble inconspicuously and let people wonder whether it is your first snack or your eighth.

On the way to the office I might stop for a donut or two, or maybe a soft-serve ice cream cone. For the sake of totals, let's say I had a couple of custard-filled donuts, common to my diet back then. They would have each been 270 calories for a total of 540, 50 percent of it fat.

So before my second meal of the day, I'm at nearly 3100 calories and 41 percent fat, not including the snacks at school. If nothing had been offered, I probably would have bought a candy bar or two, totaling more than 400 calories. For the sake of accuracy, I will not include those here.

For dinner, sometime late afternoon or early evening, I would have a fast-food meal similar to what I had for lunch, only I would go for variety, this time choosing Burger King. I would have a double Whopper with cheese, 935 calories and 59 percent fat. I would also have something "healthy," like a fish sandwich, a mere 495 calories and 45 percent fat. Instead of fries, I might go with onion rings, 302 calories, of which 51 percent came from fat. Another large soda would add 324 calories.

So, where are we now? Even if you are a compulsive overeater, you may not be able to identify with the prodigious amounts consumed by a young adult male. Still, look at this relatively. That supper would have been 2,056 more calories at 45 percent fat for a total of 5,148 and 43 percent fat. But I wasn't done.

Late at night after covering a ball game and before heading back to the office to do my writing and page layout, I would stop at Arby's for two roast beef sandwiches and a large Coke, 1,090 more calories, 30 percent from fat. My running total for the day was now 6,238 calories and 41 percent fat.

I hesitate to add, for fear of stretching the bounds of credulity, that I often added a trip to a pizza place with friends. And when I finally got home, I might treat myself to half a box of ice cream. It wouldn't surprise me if I was in the 7,500-10,000 calories-a-day range for months.

Should it have been any surprise that I was gaining several pounds a week? Later you will see how many calories it takes to gain or lose a pound, but for now suffice it to say that I started this type of gorging at about 275 pounds and was eating at a rate that would have maintained the weight of someone over 500 pounds. I could have easily become one of those saddest of cases: a person who is so huge that the body itself becomes a painful handicap and embarrassment. Most of those super heavyweights are that big not because of their eating habits but because of other physical and medical problems. And yet they must consume huge caloric quantities or their bodies would not maintain that weight.

I recall seeing someone much bigger than I and asking my father, "I don't look that bad, do I?"

"Not yet," he said quietly.

For sheer consumption, that may have been the worst period of my life. What was happening? Was I mourning a lost love? Worried about the transition to adulthood? Worried about my future? Enjoying the looser reins my parents held because of my age, despite still living at home?

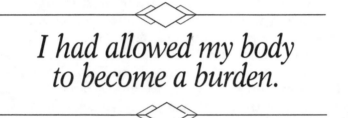

I had allowed my body to become a burden.

I was worried about my weight and had no illusions that it was skyrocketing for any reason other than my eating, but I didn't understand my compulsion to keep eating. I had the feeling that when I had had my fill of all the goodies I craved, I would start eating sensibly again and my weight would go down.

For my twentieth birthday I bought myself a new suit and thought I looked OK for a 300-plus pounder. The weight had come on so quickly that I had not yet suffered any ill effects, except for shortness of breath when going upstairs.

One night at the newspaper office I got horsing around with a couple of friends in the parking lot, and we began chasing each other between the cars. I had always taken pride in surprising people with my speed for a big person, but I had never been this big before. I found myself hardly able to move, let alone run. I tried to sprint about ten steps but felt it all over my body, particularly in my lungs and heart. What an ordeal! I huffed and puffed, not in pain but simply with the realization that I had allowed my body to become a burden. I was no longer capable of supporting it normally.

That night we went to an all-night diner, where I had two steak sandwiches and fries. I skipped the ice cream at home, but the sandwiches, along with my other fast-food intake for the day, still had me in the mega-calorie-intake category.

On my days off I also preferred fast food. I didn't know it was the salt, sugar, and fat content that was so addictive. I just liked the taste, and I enjoyed feeling full. At home I often made myself three or four peanut butter and jelly sandwiches, with butter on white bread, and washed them down with whole milk while standing at the kitchen counter.

I also enjoyed my job and my friends, though I was not dating. I began to feel lonely and unsettled about that, and when a friend began trying to interest me in a friend of his fiancée's, I was intrigued. Long before I met the girl—who is now my wife—I mentioned to my mother that I thought it was time I did something about my weight. Strangely, I recall seeing my weight as the problem, not my eating. I knew they went hand in hand, of course, but today I see the difference. The weight is just a symptom of overeating, and overeating is a symptom of a much deeper problem. In the bloom of youth and naïveté I decided to take a serious run at losing weight and didn't give much thought to the fact that I was a compulsive overeater.

My mother showed me something she had received in the mail, one of those fad diet deals that looked intriguing. I read all the promises of remarkable results and got excited and motivated. Spurred by the prospect of a new relationship, I was ready. I had my last supper, which has become a staple of most who try new diets frequently, and started the program. (I don't recall what that last supper consisted of, but it likely included my favorite burgers and desserts.)

The new program was simple, based on a balance between—of all things—foods grown above the ground and those grown below. The other two prohibitions were refined sugar and packaged or processed foods, which were said to contain all kinds of preservatives and glue that made fat stick to your body.

The thing was unscientific, of course, but it was simple and caused me to consume fewer calories. Therefore, I lost weight—and quickly. I quit eating fast food and even lost my taste for processed food. I also cut out regular soda pop and ice cream, which alone had to account for hundreds of calories each day. I ate a lot of chicken and fruit and the vegetables I liked: corn and beans. Whenever I ate anything grown below the ground, like potato or carrot, I ate three times as much of something grown above the ground, like bananas, apples, and oranges.

It all sounds pretty silly now, but I stayed away from anything that came in a package, such as breads, mixes, and the like. I would cook burgers on the grill and forgo the bun.

On the positive side, I was reminded how wonderful natural foods tasted. I have always loved fruits and many vegetables, and I came to see the other foods as the enemy. As my weight wasted away, I found the diet easy and exciting, and I was absolutely convinced I would ride this program right back down to the 200 range and stay there forever. I would simply never eat that bad stuff again.

I started the diet at about 315 pounds, or so I thought. Actually, that was all our old scale went up to, and as I look at pictures now, my guess is that I weighed closer to 330. As I melted down, the scale stayed at 315 for a while, then began dropping.

I remember an inexplicable stall at 283, which must have been an old set point (which we'll discuss later too), but then I started down again. I was still eating high quantities, sometimes dozens of chicken wings at a time, but I was eating the right things. I was no more active in sports than I had been, but I was lighter on my feet and moving more easily. Everyone noticed my thinner face and waistline.

I had met Dianna on a blind date at about 295 pounds and she was as impressed as anyone as I continued to lose. I was pleased that my weight didn't seem to bother her. You will see that over the years, her response to my private war has been most significant to my success.

In a matter of a few months I went—officially—from 315 to 256, losing almost sixty pounds. I had my clothes taken in and felt and looked better than I had in years. I was in love, and we made our wedding plans, and somewhere in there I strayed from the program. It was nothing serious. I just allowed myself a treat or two now and then.

I crept back up to 275 by the time we were married in January of 1971, but my clothes still fit, and no one would have guessed I weighed that much. I was so in love I knew I had never been in love before, and I was confident that I would not let my weight get out of hand.

We took our honeymoon traveling across the country to the southeast corner of the state of Washington, where I had accepted a job as sportswriter on a local paper. There I became active in sports again, but we also enjoyed our occasional treats at Dairy Queen. I was twenty-one years old, I was still trying to stay under 300, but I was not committed. And I didn't yet know how elusive consistency could be.

9

Getting Serious

One way I tried to stay on track when first married was to continue to avoid packaged and processed foods. I recall many meals of meat and corn, and I also recall drinking a lot of grapefruit juice—a newly acquired taste. Grapefruit juice certainly wasn't something I looked forward to, but it was supposed to be a "fat burner," and it was sure better for me than sugary soft drinks. You may recall that diet pop was pretty dreadful stuff in the early 1970s, so I didn't consider that an option.

I began to see eating the old way as a special, occasional treat. Danger. Rather than seeing such fat-laden, greasy, salty food as the poison I knew it was, it became like dessert. At the end of a long day, covering sports and writing stories, I would take Dianna out for a hoagie or a sub sandwich or some other treat that by itself would not likely have sabotaged my diet. But eating it late at night and redeveloping a taste for that type of stuff again would eventually do me in.

Such food didn't seem to bother my wife's health. She generally ate balanced meals with lots of fruits and vegetables. She was very active, enjoyed swimming, and, though she complained about five or ten pounds occasionally, seemed to have no trouble staying in shape.

A vivid memory of our slightly less than a year in Washington is that I never went out the back door of our apartment, which led to the swimming pool in the court yard. Dianna was out there nearly every day after work. Sunbathing or swimming was so foreign to me by then that I never had occasion to even venture out. To this day I couldn't even tell you the layout of the pool.

What was happening, of course, was that the occasional hoagie or sub or order of corn chips or a hot dog at a ball game began slowly and almost imperceptibly having an impact on my system. I craved that stuff and found myself thinking that it hardly made a difference in my weight. I was not gaining at the same rate I had when I was bingeing every day the year before, but slowly, a pound a week or so, the weight was coming back and the discipline unraveling.

Eventually I found myself eating both the healthy foods—to keep up appearances—and the junk food. That's a deadly combination. We sometimes think that eating healthy stuff will counteract bad eating habits, but all it does is add calories. The bad stuff far outweighs and overcomes the good. Eventually we slide back into eating only junk.

I'll spare you the details, but by spring of 1974, two job changes later, I had lost all semblance of control and was at a new peak weight. I recall a couple of attempts at reining in my weight. Once I went back to the balanced diet, swearing off packaged and processed food, eating prodigious amounts of corn and meat, and even trying jogging.

I was much too big by then to be jogging, and the most I ever ran—if you can call it that—was about four square blocks. Usually such an effort was a combination of walking and shuffling, and I always justified eating afterward. That didn't last.

I had also tried another diet. I can't even remember whether it was the Pritikin or the Scarsdale, but I do recall eating very lean meats with low-calorie catsup. I lost a few pounds in a few days and became quickly bored.

A period of successful weight loss is usually preceded by a season of frustration and even self-loathing. I experienced that for the first time early in 1974. Even when I had been gorging in 1970, I maintained some false sense of control, believing that I was choosing to eat unwisely and that I could just as easily change. But now, after a couple of short-lived efforts, I was becoming desperate.

There were a couple of evenings, after full days of work and eating, when I needed nothing else to eat. Dianna was not eating or snacking or desserting, so there was certainly no outside influence. But I found myself wanting, feeling the need, to eat more. I was stuffed but not satisfied. One night all I could find that appealed to me were oranges and milk. Imagine. The oranges tasted fine, and drinking milk with them reminded me of the kinds of lunches I enjoyed while working construction right out of high school.

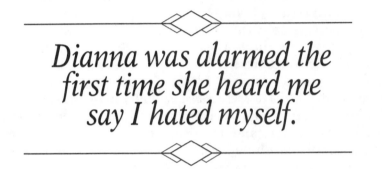

Dianna was alarmed the first time she heard me say I hated myself.

But I had not been physically hungry, so the oranges and milk simply lay on my stomach and made me uncomfortable. The acid upset my system, and I was not comfortable even sitting on the couch. By now I was well over 300 pounds and often found myself short of breath even when not exerting.

Dianna reports that I slept fitfully, constantly moving, breathing heavily, my cardiovascular system trying to service a body too big for its engine. During the day I enjoyed my work and my colleagues. I was a funny and fun-loving guy. I could poke fun at myself, and somehow I was still growing and excelling in my writing and editing. But at home, in private, I was miserable.

Dianna was alarmed the first time she heard me say I hated myself. I hadn't allowed myself to even think that in the past. But I was so frustrated at continuing to eat even when I was stuffed and knew better that I felt like a failure. What was wrong with me? Had I tried to get to the root of *that*, rather than simply trying to diet, I might have headed off a lifetime of self-induced pain. But I couldn't see past my own self-destructive eating, so the only solution was to get serious about it and do something.

Getting ready to seriously diet, for me at least, is something that builds. It comes on gradually as I get more and more disgusted with myself and dissatisfied with my life. You have heard, and maybe have yourself said, "I've got to do something about this soon." I've learned that such statements signal a good, healthy time in the life of a compulsive overeater. If I've learned nothing else over the years, I've learned that outside motivation is virtually worthless, short-lived at best. Inward motivation is the only hope.

I was getting there. I was tired of the way I felt, tired of the way my clothes fit, tired of the way I looked in the mirror and—even worse—the way I looked in pictures. Why is it that we can actually fool ourselves occasionally in the mirror? Maybe we have learned to turn a certain way, or smile a certain way, or look only at our eyes and hair. But a camera will not be fooled. You get those snapshots back, and though you are dressed up and smiling, that body seems to dominate everything and everybody. You're twice the size of anyone else in the picture. That belly seems never-ending. Even your shoulders and neck are bulging. Your eyes are tiny slits peeking out of huge cheeks. Your fingers are fat, your knuckles dimply like a baby's. And you know that all those people who have said, "You're not really fat; you're just big" are really lying, just as you have been lying to yourself.

I had gone past the point where I could camouflage it anymore. I was a big, fat guy, out of shape, unhealthy, undisciplined. No stories about my damaged metabolism or my childhood heart disease could explain away my weight and my fat, and soon I got to the place where I didn't want to try to explain it away.

I was ready to get serious, and I began looking for a solution.

Weight Watchers was one of the most popular programs back then, and rightfully still is. It was inexpensive, and from what I had heard about it, it seemed like something I could handle. I was past looking for a starvation diet. I had proven I could be successful by changing *what* I ate rather than *how much*, and from the Weight Watcher literature I had seen, it looked sensible and balanced.

The local group met in the basement of a church. After a last supper (this time consisting of steaks and ice cream), I went alone, signed up, paid up, and weighed in. Even I was surprised. I was up to 330 pounds. I had known I was over 300, but I didn't know how much. The scale at home didn't go that high.

I loved Weight Watchers. Our leader was a woman who had lost more than sixty pounds and had kept it off for five years. She was funny, articulate, encouraging, and supportive. Best of all, the group of a hundred or so was made up almost entirely of women, most of them my mother's age. I don't know why, but I thought that was great! Many of them were shy and old-fashioned. They were polite and friendly, and they were glad to have a young man in the group.

A couple of older guys were there because of their diabetes or some other ailment. About half the group were hanging on, trying to maintain losses they had racked up in previous weeks. But the other half seemed to be succeeding, either losing or maintaining.

Best of all, Weight Watchers had that silly little ritual of applauding anyone who had lost weight during the week. Not much was said about anyone who had gained, unless they chose to volunteer that news and ask questions. But if you had lost even as little as a quarter of a pound, you were applauded by the rest of the group.

Now, think of it. Here I was, a third child, irrationally starved for attention despite the love and support of my family, my wife, and even my colleagues, still subconsciously trying to please my parents. And here was a roomful of women my mother's age! When I lost weight, they applauded!

Let me clarify again: whatever need I had for my parents' approval was not due to any lack of effort on their part. I do not say that simply to make them feel better. Anyone who knows them knows they love me and are proud of me and have always supported me unconditionally. But over the years, as I have tried to get a handle on my own needs and weaknesses, I still sense a striving within to prove myself. It's my problem, not theirs, but you can see how the Weight Watchers format was so appealing to me.

Well, there's no genteel way to tell you: I was a Weight Watchers superstar. I lost so much so fast that I occasionally got *standing* ovations. I realize that my initial loss was astounding partly because of that last supper, which probably added three to five pounds of water weight alone, but get this: the first week on Weight Watchers, carefully following their program for men (which included four pieces of bread and five fruits a day, along with all the other normal, balanced foods), I lost seventeen and a half pounds!

I knew I had lost at least ten, but seventeen and a half! I quickly became known to all in the group, and week after week they waited to hear how I had done. The second week I lost another three pounds, and that was my smallest loss in the first ten weeks or so. In just fifteen weeks I lost 88.5 pounds and melted from 330 to 242.5.

One of the great advantages of that program, in my mind, is that the foods are normal. I combined them and manipulated them. For instance, I was religious about weighing my food and remaining very strict for breakfast. I ate the lighter, high-air content cereals that looked like more, despite their weight. If I got an ounce of cereal with skim milk, I made sure it was Rice Krispies, because they looked so voluminous in the bowl.

I would also have one of my five fruits for breakfast, maybe an orange. I think I substituted a piece of bread for something later in the day so I could have a slice of toast too. So a small, satisfying breakfast left me hungry for lunch.

Lunch was the greatest. It was as if I wasn't even on a diet. I had carefully measured out my allotted ounces of chicken and my tablespoon of mayonnaise, used my four remaining slices of bread, and added lettuce for two (count 'em) chicken sandwiches. I could have all the noncaloric drinks I wanted, and as I wasn't a coffee and tea drinker, water or diet pop were my only options. The diet colas were still pretty dreadful, so I opted for Diet 7-Up. A sixteen-ounce bottle with the sandwiches, an apple, and an orange was a very big lunch for anyone.

To me it was almost like cheating! I was eating well and eating a lot—though considerably less than I had before—and I was wasting away.

I don't recall my dinners well, but I do know that I cheated on the program. Our leader would gently scold me for admitting that, but every week people asked for advice, and they wanted to hear from me. Here I was, doing something right. After my ovation, they would also boo and hiss lovingly because of my metabolism. The leader would try to put my loss in perspective because of my maleness, my youth, my activity level, and all that, but the fact remained: this was a program made for me.

But when people said, "Do you cheat? How do you keep from sneaking what you shouldn't have? I can't stay away from this or that," I had an answer: Cheat *on* the program, not *off* it. I meant simply that when you must have something to eat, have more of what the program allowed. In other words, I might have more than the allotted five fruits a day (women were allowed three back then). If I was truly hungry, I might have three or four or even more apples in addition to my daily allotment.

Again, our leader always said that sticking to the program was the best way, but it was hard to argue with someone who was averaging losses of more than five pounds a week.

Needless to say, that was one of the headiest times of my life. I was twenty-four, I had been married three years, had a new job, a new body, and a new outlook. I didn't know why my weight loss programs had not lasted in the past, but surely this one would. Why in the world would anyone with a new lease on life, who had proved he could lose, not continue right on down to the 220s and stay there forever?

Why, indeed?

10

Yo-Yo City

My intentions were the best. The rapid weight loss had been so invigorating that I drank in all the accolades. I had not even thought of exercising, though I found myself more mobile than ever. Once, at a picnic, I had to jog across a bridge to find someone, and I couldn't believe how light I felt. My legs had developed tremendous strength over the years, carrying all that excess weight. Now that the weight was gone, the muscle remained, and I felt as if I were flying. I actually had to slow down to maintain my balance.

Because of my youth and the relatively short time that I had been so heavy, my skin had enough elasticity that I was not left with sagging excess, despite the speed of my loss. My abdomen was flat, my face taut. Most people guessed my weight at about 190. I looked taller than 6'1".

I never considered myself particularly good-looking, and still don't, but it had been years since I noticed women glancing at me without immediately looking away.

What a thrill it was to buy normal-sized clothes! I never tired of the compliments over my new look. Best of all, Dianna did not overreact. She was happy and proud of me, but nothing she did or said implied that she loved me any more or less depending on my size. I knew she wanted me alive and healthy, but I was also confident that her love did not hinge on my weight.

I remember the first small bag of M&Ms that was the beginning of the end for me. I don't blame my failure on Weight Watchers or their program. As I've said, any legitimate weight loss program that includes balanced meals, fiber, and the right vitamins and nutrients is to be commended and will work. When we fail, it's because we don't stay with it. How or why we fall off the program should not be laid at the feet of those who invented the program.

Weight Watchers was big on not calling their system a diet. It was a program, a lifestyle. There was even a lot of talk about avoiding that old trap of thinking, *Once I'm finished with the program, I'll . . .* whatever. Unfortunately, unless that is really drilled in, that's how we all think, isn't it? Once I'm off this diet, I'll work in some of those things I've been missing.

I tried to tell myself I wouldn't do that, and for a long time I didn't. But at one point, after getting down to 242.5, I was driving back to work after lunch one day and got a hankering for something sweet. I wanted some M&M peanuts, and I went through a lot of mental gymnastics to talk myself into them. Today I would say, fine, go ahead, have them, but make sure they fit into your day's total calories and fat percentages. Then you won't binge. Or you shouldn't.

As I look back on it, three things contributed to my failure to maintain that weight loss, and one of them has nothing to do with how quickly I lost it. I know that the faster you lose the harder it is to maintain, but for me I firmly believe that was not the case. I needed the quick loss to stay motivated. But, first, I was a perfectionist; second, I never kept a food diary; and, third, I did not exercise. Nothing sounded less interesting to me than working out, and, whereas keeping a diary was encouraged, it was not required. Exercise was discussed but not emphasized the way it is today. I didn't think I needed either. I'll discuss the hopelessness of perfectionism later.

Back then, an M&M lapse was major. Deep in the back of my mind I had a feeling that I was violating some carefully designed law. Perhaps from my Christian upbringing I equated a candy treat as the first step down a slippery slope of failure.

I convinced myself that wouldn't happen, that I would simply enjoy the treat and forget it. But I told no one. I bought my candy at a gas station, enjoyed it (not as much as I thought I would; isn't that always so?), and otherwise stayed on the program.

Of course, a couple of ounces of candy one day in an otherwise solid week not only will not adversely affect your weight or your diet, but *can* also actually keep you from failing in a larger way. But I didn't know that. To weigh in the next week and find that I had not gained was a great boost. I had, in essence, gotten away with the candy.

And so the next week I had some ice cream.

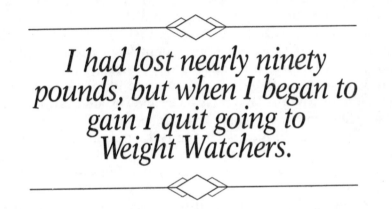

I had lost nearly ninety pounds, but when I began to gain I quit going to Weight Watchers.

You know what happened next. As my perfectionism gave way to cheating, my weight stuck or started to rise a little. I started wearing less and less to weigh-ins. Good thing it was summer. Within a few weeks I was down to a T-shirt and beltless shorts. It was then that I noticed that everyone else had done the same.

From the beginning I had determined to weigh in with my shoes on and in a normal outfit. Now at least five of the pounds not showing up on the scale were in my shoes and clothes. I didn't stay around through the winter to see what people did then. They must have come hardly dressed under their warm coats and boots.

Our Weight Watcher teacher noticed that my weight had stalled. She also noticed that I often skipped the meeting if my weigh-in showed I'd gained. She encouraged me to stay with it, to not skip weigh-ins and classes. She said that there often seems to be a barrier as a person gets close to a hundred-pound loss, which had been my goal. But I was no longer getting applause. No one expressed concern, but suddenly I was no longer the star. Others had joined, and they were losing, and I was clapping for them.

Depressed over a slight gain, I would stop on the way home for ice cream, telling myself that I had a whole week to lose whatever it added. A few days later, after a few more treats, I told myself I still had three or four more days, if I really deprived myself. Deprivation was not at the heart of the program and had never worked for me.

My clothes still fit and I was still trying very hard to hang on. I continued to get encouragement from friends and relatives, but I felt like a fraud. I had lost nearly ninety pounds, but when I began to gain I quit going to Weight Watchers. If I occasionally saw the Weight Watcher lady around town, I would assure her that I was "going to get back into it." Have you ever used that phrase? When we're unraveling, coming out the other side of a good weight loss and know we're losing control, that's what we say. "I've got to regroup, get serious again, get back into it, start over."

A job I had dreamed about for a long time, editor of *Moody* magazine (then called *Moody Monthly*) opened up, and I was recommended for it. I pursued it with vigor and was thrilled to be selected. It meant a big change in our lives because, now, rather than leaving home fifteen minutes before work and getting home for lunch and then fifteen minutes after work, I would be leaving at the crack of dawn for Chicago and returning early in the evening. We didn't have children yet, but Dianna and I were used to more time together.

We decided that the ministry opportunity and challenge were worth it, and we devised ways to keep our relationship strong. I did, however, find the new job distracting to my diet—another common excuse for straying from a program. By the time I started working at Moody in October of 1974, I had turned twenty-five and was back up to about 265 pounds. I was still wearing the new clothes I had purchased after the big loss, though they were getting tight. That made me feel fatter than I was and more of a failure—and a rather immediate one at that.

On the staff at Moody I met a new friend who had recently lost a hundred pounds and was beginning to put it back on. We were not good for each other during the few months we worked together. We tried to help each other, but when one was weak the other was also. We both enjoyed the same kinds of foods, and when we got in the mood we enjoyed them together. I tell the following story for its humor, and yet it is also sad.

We had both been very good on our diets for about a week; our wives had packed us healthy lunches of chicken and veggies. I had, however, already begun skipping breakfast again. One morning I popped my head into my friend's office and said ruefully, "What did you get in your bag today?"

He showed me his slices of meat and his fruit, and I showed him my healthy stuff. "What do you say we eat these for breakfast and enjoy a good lunch today?" To my shame, this was my idea. He quickly agreed. We wolfed down our lunches at about eight in the morning.

At break someone had a birthday party. We had already planned to blow off the day, so we indulged in cake and ice cream. Of course, we were not really hungry for lunch an hour and a half later, but we had been looking forward to it all day. It became a progressive lunch.

We started across the street to a greasy spoon that specialized in burgers and Polish sausage. We had one of each, with fries and a large Coke. We were stuffed. But, we wondered, were these burgers and these Polish really better than at the two places down the street, one of which specialized in burgers and the other in sausages?

We moved down the street and tried the specialty at each place. By then we weren't tasting much, but we made our judgments and waddled back toward Moody. After all that salt and fat and grease, we needed (why, of course we did) something sweet. We stopped at the Divine Ice Cream Shoppe, which, strangely enough, did not have ice cream but rather specialized in donuts. We each had two raised glazed.

Now we were in serious pain. But we had had a taste for ice cream. So on our way back to our offices, we stopped in the Coffee Cove downstairs for an ice cream bar. I wish I could say it really hit the spot. But by now neither of us was pretending this was even funny anymore, and, because we were basically good guys, we encouraged each other not to let all that fat and sugar keep us from putting in a full day's work for a full day's pay.

In the afternoon I was feeling pretty logy as I slogged through my work, but I forced myself to finish a couple of projects before I made my way down the hall to see how my friend was doing. I knocked and entered his office, only to see him quickly shut his desk drawer and stop chewing in midbite. He grinned sheepishly, and I saw the telltale orange signs of Cheetos around his mouth. "Hey," I said, accusingly, "give me some of those."

We laughed and polished off that bag and decided we could never do this again. We wouldn't really need to eat again for a week. But now for the greatest irony of all: our wives had run into each other in the grocery store that very day and shared their pride and admiration over how their respective husbands had been doing on their diets for several days. They agreed it would be a good idea to reward us with our favorite dinners. They would still not compromise us with ice cream and gravies and all that, but these would be feasts nonetheless.

I don't remember what *his* favorite meal was, but *I* was treated to a pork roast with all the trimmings. I forced it down, unable to admit—then—what I had done. When my wife told me why she was doing that and that my friend was enjoying the same treat at his home, I could hardly keep a straight face. I'd like to say we learned our lessons.

Despite my poor track record, I never gave up. For a while I resigned myself to the fact that I had been a failure, but months later, when my weight got back up to about 313 and felt like 350, I swallowed my pride and headed back to Weight Watchers. (After another last supper, of course.)

This time I took some friends from work, and we all tried it together. I lost nine pounds the first week, was disappointed, and soon began to unravel again. Now I was really discouraged. I was frustrated and felt unmotivated. I tried to come up with all kinds of rationalizations and excuses, but I knew they didn't hold water.

Once I was off the program, and no longer pretending I was still trying, my weight began to skyrocket again. At this point, I never saw my dilemma as a spiritual problem. I prayed for help, but I never did my part. I believed that the Lord would remind me —when I prayed and asked Him to—that I didn't really need the extra food, that I could turn it down, and that I would be glad I did. But when He reminded me, I disobeyed. I didn't hold it against God that He didn't supernaturally keep me from eating. I never prayed that I would lose my desire or love for food. I sensed that wasn't the real problem. I simply wasn't succeeding.

One night I sat battling the urge to have some potato chips, after I had had a good, sensible dinner and needed nothing else. I sat on the couch, warring with myself, went to the kitchen, looked at the bag, and won the battle. I remember going back to the living room, without having succumbed to the temptation, and feeling a real sense of victory.

Nowhere in the back of my mind did I have the idea that I would have to fight the same battle half an hour later. If I had, and had I been serious, I would have tossed those chips or put them where I couldn't get at them, or told Dianna that I didn't want them in the house. But why should I deprive her of a treat she knew how to handle?

The strangest thing was that when I went resolutely to the kitchen later and indulged in those chips, I saw the two incidents as totally separate. And they were. The fact that I eventually broke down and "cheated" in no way negated the victory I had scored earlier. Had I resisted the first time, knowing full well I would eat them later, the victory would have been hollow. But I maintain that that had been a real success, even though I eventually failed. In a peculiar way, it was a major step for me. I realized that I could win, I could succeed, and then I might face the same battle again and again.

As I neared a point of self-loathing once more, the rest of my life seemed to be in perfect order. I was appreciated at Moody and my work was recognized and rewarded. I had begun writing books on the side and seemed to have all the work I wanted and needed. Dianna and I were in the foundational stages of a wonderful marriage. And best of all, she was expecting.

When Dallas came along, July 25, 1975, I was nearing another crisis. I knew it was time to take another serious run at losing weight. If being responsible for a new life wasn't motivation enough, I didn't know what was.

It would be nearly another year before I decided on what route to go this time, and my last supper would consist of deep dish Chicago-style pizza and mint chip ice cream. But I had the feeling that this time had to be the last time. I didn't want to be one of those statistics, a victim of yo-yo dieting that resulted in more trouble than just staying fat.

I was desperate—and down to what I considered my last chance.

11

The Last Chance Diet

Desperate people do desperate things.

I was still looking for a key, an easy answer. Nothing had worked, and I was not yet willing to admit that it was I who had not worked. I had tried. I had been determined. I thought I had done my best. But I didn't allow myself to become one of those who said this or that program didn't work for me.

All the programs work if you follow them correctly and stick with them. But in my frantic search, I found one that might have succeeded in doing me real damage had I stuck with it long enough.

I read a book called *The Last Chance Diet*, which told of a new idea. It called for a lengthy all-liquid fast consisting mainly of protein powder mixed with water, taken three or four times a day. From this you would get all your vitamins and nutrients, except those provided in supplemental capsules. Other than that, you were to eat or drink nothing except noncaloric liquids.

There was something frightening and exciting about this prospect. The decisions would be made for you. It wasn't a matter of what or how much, it was a matter of simply doing what you were told. The book carefully outlined the possible side effects, the difficulty of getting through the first few days, the headaches, the hunger pangs, all that.

I was intrigued. I was willing to try anything and to stay on it for however many months it would take to get down to under 200 pounds. That alone, I believed, would be enough motivation to keep me on track for the rest of my life.

I thought about this for a long time, but I didn't know where or how to begin. Then I happened to find an article on the same plan in one of my wife's women's magazines. At the end it listed various doctors across the country who monitored such programs. What could be better than that? It would be expensive, but no more expensive than food.

The basic premise was that, as the body looks for energy and doesn't find it because of the hyper-low calories, it begins to feed on itself in a process called ketosis. It's auto-cannibalism (the body burns its own fat reserves), and it provides quick weight loss. No way I would want to try that without medical supervision.

I looked up the doctor in the Chicago area who was a proponent of that kind of weight loss. His staff was friendly and personable, and they ran me through a long series of tests and questionnaires to determine my suitability for the program. I felt as if I were auditioning, but I knew I would qualify. I weighed more than enough, and I'd had a history of frustration.

One of the more distasteful parts of the test was for glucose tolerance. After several hours of not eating or drinking, I was given what I can only describe as the equivalent of straight cola syrup. It was thick and strong and sweet. After I'd taken that and eliminated, the urine was tested.

I was also weighed (327) and measured and had my fat sized up with calipers by a quiet young woman with "M.D." after the name on her nameplate. The coordinator of the program, a wavy-haired man in a white coat who wore a name bracelet, explained that he was the only person in the office who was not an M.D. or an R.N. He informed me that my heart tests showed "right bundle branch blockage," which sounded an awful lot like a serious cardiac disease. My blood was also high in triglycerides and fat. I was the perfect candidate, and they would be happy to welcome me into the program.

I began enthusiastically. Their "beverage," such as it was, came in vanilla, chocolate, and strawberry. The only one I could stomach was the chocolate, and all three had that powdery protein smell I can hardly endure today. I had to plug my nose when I drank it, and I shuddered with the yuckiness of it.

But I was religious about the program. They gave me a weekly shot with an appetite suppressant, which I believe worked. I quickly tired of forcing down the liquid and the capsules, but I did get to the point where I looked forward to those drinks, distasteful as they were.

I lost a little over ten pounds the first week, and I desperately needed affirmation. I had endured the lowest psychological hours of my life, mourning the loss of food, feeling despair at not being able to look forward to meals, wondering if I had done the right thing, wondering if this all made sense. I was beginning to hear stories of people who had died on similar programs and of probes by government officials into just this type of weight control.

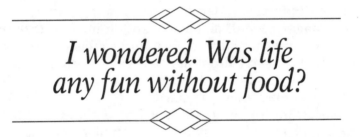

I wondered. Was life any fun without food?

When I saw the program coordinator at my first weigh-in I proudly told him that I had not cheated and that I had lost more than ten pounds. (I have since learned that the likely reason the loss was less than it had been on Weight Watchers was that the fast was such a shock to my system that my body clearly tried to protect itself from starvation.)

Compare the reaction I got from the office manager to the applause I got at Weight Watchers: "Is that all? We have women losing more than that! Are you sure you didn't cheat?"

I was sure. I was miserable. During the second week of the program people began to notice my new demeanor. I could not smile. My thighs were disappearing, my stomach was going down, my face lost its puffiness, but I was emotionally flat. People asked me if it was worth it. I wondered. Was life any fun without food? I told myself this was temporary.

My beverage powder mix came in Tupperware containers, my vitamin capsules in clear plastic bags. I had never seen the doctor whose name was on the door. But I was losing weight, and that was what I wanted.

I was obsessed with food. One of the roads on my way home had fast-food places on either side for miles. Every sign worked on me, every smell. I found myself noticing every word in conversation that was food related or even rhymed with something food related. When people used expressions such as "a piece of cake" or "easy as pie," my hunger was triggered. I was acutely aware of the impact of TV advertising on our appetites.

I wanted to smell everyone's food. When I sat at a meal, I would urge people to slow down and enjoy it, to not leave any, to savor every bite. I'm sure they got tired of me real quickly as I sat there sipping ice water with lemon wedges in it.

Our magazine staff had a convention in New York, an international center for cuisine. I sat and watched them eat Italian one night, nearly drooling. In a cafe I was so obnoxious about a colleague's bacon, lettuce, and tomato sandwich that he had to give me a silencing stare.

Alone in my room, at the appointed times, I mixed my beverage and forced it down. It eventually became a little more palatable, but not much. The headaches had left me, and I was not physically hungry, but mouth hunger and psychological hunger were still problems. I was depressed, down, restless. The fast weight loss was encouraging, but I felt no support from the doctor's office. They took my money, but they didn't seem to care. I had to pass a charcoal-burger place right next to the doctor's office, and it was no fun to pass up. It was all I could do to look straight ahead on weigh-in day as I headed back to my car.

An upcoming business trip to Bermuda would allow Dianna and me a week together in a beautiful spot. I was two weeks into the Last Chance Diet when I got there, and I thought the new setting would make my deprivation easier.

It was torture.

The first night our hosts invited magazine executives from all over the U.S. to a cookout on the ocean shore. Under swaying palms in the warm summer breeze they cooked pork and beef and chicken over hardwood. It was one of the most delicious looking (and smelling) feasts I have ever seen. To make matters worse, I found myself away from the hotel and my beverage supply during my usual time for my last dose of the day. So I was actually hungry and undernourished as I sat with my wife and hundreds of others who were enjoying those goodies.

That had to be the toughest time of all. I drank ice water and watched people eat my favorite foods, cooked my favorite, succulent way, in a setting so beautiful it could make you cry. And it almost did.

There was also fresh baked bread, beans, coleslaw. Well, I could go on. From a culinary point of view, that was one of the low lights of my life, having to pass up that wonderful stuff. But I did it, and when I finally got back to the hotel I snarfed down my drink quickly and went to bed unhappy. I should have felt a great sense of accomplishment, and Dianna tried to encourage me. She couldn't believe I had endured, and she said she wouldn't have blamed me or thought less of me if I had not. But she was amazed and proud of me.

What worried me was the lack of pride I felt in that woeful experience and something playing at the edges of my brain. However tenuous my resolve from the beginning of the program, it was beginning to unwind. I could just feel it.

The night before we were to leave Bermuda, we were on our own for dinner. I didn't think I could handle another experience like the first night. I had sat watching my wife and others eat at lunches and dinners the other days as well, so Dianna and I decided that she would simply order room service, which she would eat while I read or watched television.

Had I known I was going to fall off the program that night and finish her meal of scallops, a leftover roll, and half her dessert, I would have cashed it in the first night and enjoyed what I really wanted: all that great meat cooked over wood in the open air.

The stuff I enjoyed in the room that night was OK, but it wasn't the ecstatic experience I expected after twenty days of fasting. Seafood was all right with me but had never been a favorite. I was stunned at how casually and quickly I went over the edge, once I allowed myself the luxury.

You may wonder at Dianna's reaction. I have to say it was perfect. During my entire adult battle with food, she couldn't have been better. Call it boorishness or selfishness or oversensitivity, but I am one of those who would react totally inappropriately if my wife felt it was her place to badger me, criticize me, coach me, remind me, put me on diets, or anything of the sort.

I don't know why exactly, but any hint that she was as disappointed in me as I was in myself would have sent me into a major tailspin. I would not blame her, of course, but I could see myself regressing rather than progressing in my resolve and discipline if I thought her love and respect hinged on my discipline.

Whenever I was losing weight, someone was sure to ask Dianna, "Was this your idea? Did you put him on this diet?" I was always gratified that she made clear that she wasn't about to even suggest such a thing. From day one she has maintained that my weight is my personal business and that no one can do anything about it but me.

She has always been careful, when we talk about it, to acknowledge that she obviously wants me healthy, happy, comfortable, and at peace with myself. Her unspoken message is the same as the only one that ever seems to work with an alcoholic: "I know you can do it, and when you're ready, I'll be here to support you in any way you wish."

She has never said, "Oh, no, you don't want to fall off your program now, after you've done so well." She doesn't even give me a startled look or a raised eyebrow. If I had lost fifty pounds and told her as she left for the grocery store that I wanted some ice cream, she wouldn't even bat an eye. She would simply ask, "What flavor?"

There are those, I know, who consider this enabling behavior. Believe me, in my case, it is not. I know my eating behavior is wrong and that it is an ugly trait. But if she gave me any of those reactions, I would become defensive and angry and would feel judged. Irrationally (I know) I would feel that her love and acceptance were conditional.

Rather, I thrive on her confidence. Even when I ask, "Do I want a brownie?" or, "Should I have some pie with the rest of you?" as opposed to eating an apple, she merely says—and means—"It's up to you."

Though I am immature and stunted in this area, she treats me like an adult rather than a child. When I am, in essence, asking her permission, it may appear that I need to be told, "No, as long as you're asking, that is precisely what you don't want to do." Rather, she is putting the responsibility right back where it belongs. She's saying, without judgment, "This is your thing, not mine. You do what you're going to do."

Often, simply knowing that she is not going to be parental about it causes me to make the right decision. Now, were she truly an enabler, she would say, "Go ahead, enjoy. You've been good long enough. One little piece of cake won't hurt you." You can see how much better it is for my psyche and my well-being that she simply supports me, wherever I happen to be in my resolve.

Of course, I get positive strokes when I'm strong. She often tells me, "I knew you could do it. You can do anything you set your mind to. You've been stronger than I ever would have been on this program."

On the other hand, her neutral reactions when I am doing something stupid makes it impossible for me to pass the blame, much as we compulsive overeaters like to do. Do you ever find yourself saying, "Why did you buy that? Why did you leave that out? Why did you let me have that?"

This cuts both ways. If I don't want her telling me what to do or not do in this area, I can't blame her when I do what I want. When I have asked her not to bake my favorite cookies a day or two into a new resolve, she always obliges. And she never simply brings me a treat unbidden, because I am the type who will likely not refuse it.

If there's a perfect wife for a man with my problem, I have her. Though there are those who say she should be confrontive and scold me and insist that I stay healthy for her sake and the sake of the kids, I say that would imply that I don't have the same goals and feel just as bad when I fail.

Ironically, because her own weight problem is only in her own mind (a few pounds now and then), she is the opposite.

She wants me to remind her, to "not let" her have a dessert, to ask her if she "really wants" something. I was slow to pick up on that and refused to do it for many years because I know how it would bug me. But when she asked me to do it and I didn't and she failed, she would say, "Why didn't you tell me not to have that?"

I'd say, "Do you really want me to?"

She insisted that she did, and so when we were out and someone offered a dessert, I would decline and she would get that "thinking about it" smile and look to me for support. All I could force myself to say was, "Are you going to regret it?" And she would pass it up too. I confess, that same message coming the other way would make me accept the dessert and, of course, still hate myself later.

Before I tell the rest of my Last Chance Diet story, let me just say this if you are the spouse of someone waging the weight war:

Regardless of your tack over the years, you will do well to resolve to be unconditionally loving and supportive. It doesn't seem to make sense, and given the slight possibility that your overeating spouse might react positively to badgering or parenting, you might at least want to have a frank discussion about it sometime.

But my prediction is—and you should give your spouse a chance to corroborate this and then be prepared to act upon it —that a totally nonjudgmental approach will reap more benefits in the long run.

It won't be easy. You may resolve to never say another critical thing, never give one look of disapproval. You may even say and mean with all your heart, "Honey, if you gain a hundred pounds, I won't love you any less." But when your spouse starts to gain, it will be painful for you. You'll feel like an enabler. You'll wonder if you haven't "given permission" for this unhealthy slide.

Yet, when your spouse is convinced you're serious, that you know he or she can do it, light will appear at the end of their tunnel. The only time, in my experience, that a fat person is ready for input is when he brings up the subject. Even then, your response is critical.

If your spouse says, "I hate myself. I can't get a handle on this. I have to do something about it. I'm tried of being fat and feeling like a failure. I have no control, etc., etc., etc.," that's the time to carefully make your points:

"I'm sorry it's so hard for you. I can tell how painful it is for you. You know I love you just the way you are. Don't feel you have to do this for me. Whenever you're ready, I'll support whatever you want to do about it. Tell me what to say or do or not say or not do."

And when your spouse says anything about embarrassing you with the way he or she looks or how disappointed you must be or how you could have had a thin and in-shape spouse, that is a dire time. Before giving a flippant answer, think in advance what you're going to say. Don't lie. Don't say, "You don't look that bad."

Determine in your own mind and heart that outward appearance is less important and be able to say that in all honesty. What your spouse wants to hear right then is an expression of unconditional love. "I love you just the way you are. I'm proud you're mine. I don't want you to be unhappy, but don't think I'll love you less either way."

As irrational as it sounds, and even though you may feel as if you are not contributing to the effort to lose weight and get healthier, trust me—you are doing the most positive thing you can. At some point, go over this advice with your spouse and see if he or she doesn't agree. If your spouse doesn't, then speak frankly about what you can do that will be the most helpful.

I have heard horror stories of spouses asking each other, "What are you going to do about your weight?" And when one complains, "I'm gaining," the other says, "Quit eating so much."

Call it sin, call it slovenliness, call it selfishness, call it irrational, but the spouse with the problem will spiral into more self-destructive behavior. He or she will eat in secret, get depressed because of a sense of conditional love, and whatever well-intentioned goal you had in mind will never be realized.

As in my case, your spouse may be failing on a last chance diet.

12

Desperation

Despite my perfectionistic tendencies—which usually caused me to fall off the wagon as soon as I'd had a setback on a diet—I somehow recovered from that lapse in Bermuda and got back on the program immediately the next day. I was back to the yucky beverage, ignored the tasty-looking little meal on the airplane, avoided all the fast-food joints, and was able to fairly easily get back into fasting gear.

That surprised me, because the early headaches and the niggling depression did not return. Maybe I felt good that I could rebound, but it didn't last long. I enjoyed another significant weight loss the next week, and at the end of thirty days, despite the one lapse, I had lost thirty pounds.

And then one day I lost it. You may know the feeling. You simply get it into your head that you are going to eat what you want and nothing will deter you. You can sit and count to ten, you can call a friend, you can pray, you can talk to yourself, but you're headed toward disaster and you know it.

I had had my beverage in the morning, my pills midmorning, and even my noon beverage. I was a full ten days past the Bermuda failure, but I had many months yet to go on the fast. It suddenly loomed too large a task, and, as I headed toward the refrigerator, I had a feeling this was the end. I said something to Dianna about blowing the day off, as if this would be another temporary lapse, but I believe I knew better. I was playing a mind game with myself, but I was a veteran at this stuff by now.

In the refrigerator freezer were some Reese's Peanut Butter Cups, a favorite of mine. Now, note—when I am psyched in, even my favorite stuff cannot tempt me. To this day, simply being a day or two in advance of weigh-in is enough to motivate me to walk past freshly baked goodies. Wave a frosted brownie under my nose when I am zoned in, and you only make me proud to show off my resolve.

But when resolve is unraveling, there's nothing like an old favorite that slides down quickly. I made quick work of the Peanut Butter Cups, and the ice cream wasn't far behind. I was careful enough not to make myself sick, knowing that the calories and sugar alone were enough of a shock to my system without adding the stretching of my fragile stomach.

When I weighed in the next day and still saw a loss, I had the idea that I might get back on track. And yet, didn't I have six days to make up for another indulgence, like one of those burgers next door, the ones I had passed up every time?

I stopped in, ordered one, and watched them make it. I did worry that someone from the doctor's office might see me in there, but, on the other hand, they had again taken my smaller-than-normal weight loss in stride. Maybe they thought I was past the initial, big-loss stage and that this was normal. There was no counseling, no therapy, no group support, and little enthusiasm. I was still getting my supplies in Tupperware containers and plastic bags, and I still had never met the doctor.

This burger was going to be good. And it was. I ate it slowly and savored it, telling myself it was the last treat that week. But of course it wasn't. Once the door is open, things get in and out that were not intended.

Ironically, at church the next week a woman who was a major distributor of weight control products and supplements through one of the household-product–pyramid-selling programs asked me crassly what I was doing about my weight. I told her about the program, and she said I could save money and get the stuff just as easily through her. I told her I was trying to be more careful by going through a doctor. But when I told her his name, she was shocked.

"Why, he's been winning national awards for months for distributing the same thing I'm distributing! He's doing this through his medical practice?" I nodded.

"That's against the rules, and it wouldn't surprise me if it's illegal."

I didn't think much more about it, but that explained the Tupperware and the plastic bags. This was no medical or scientific thing; it was a guy cashing in on a sales scheme. No wonder I had never seen him! He was probably off to the Far East on some trip he had won or was out fishing on the boat he had won.

At the same time dire stories appeared in the press about people dying on the very program I was on. What a handy excuse to get off it! I was already cheating and feeling terrible, just when people were starting to notice my weight loss, but here was a ready-made reason to actually protect my health by getting off this dangerous program.

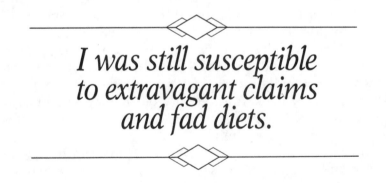

I was still susceptible to extravagant claims and fad diets.

Though I needed no other reason, one day an official car from the State of Illinois pulled into my driveway and an agent asked if he could chat with me for a few minutes about my doctor. I was on my way somewhere, but I sensed that this was more important. The man was with a state regulating agency, and he knew a lot more about me and my experience than I did. But I was able to corroborate his suspicions and findings.

I confirmed that the beverage was being sold over the counter at the office as medical treatment. He probed my memory of the screening process and asked whether, like other patients, I had never met the doctor but was assured by the program coordinator that he was the only non-M.D. on the staff. All true, I told him, and then he told *me* a few things.

The people with M.D. after their names were not even R.N.s. The people giving me injections were just office personnel. The doctor was a lazy, greedy guy in deep trouble. Later, I read in the paper that he eventually evaded prosecution and incarceration by surrendering his medical license.

What I learned from all that, I don't know, except that I would never again be quite so cavalier about entering into a program just because it had the trappings of credibility. For many years after that, all-liquid fasts were in disrepute, and I spoke as a bit of an expert on the dangers. The fact was, I had failed on the program, but I wondered if I might have done more severe damage to my system had I been able to stay on it.

Believe it or not, there were benefits to having endured that fast. I appreciated food more than ever. I stopped eating between meals so that I could enjoy a modicum of hunger. (Someone has said that hunger is the best seasoning.) So I was less of a snacker and more of a healthy eater. But because I was still occasionally a compulsive overeater, my weight was destined to come back. And because of the way I had lost it—quickly and drastically, losing muscle mass as well as fat—I was predisposed to gain quickly.

At one point I was invited to an Overeaters Anonymous meeting and introduced myself as a compulsive overeater. As soon as I said it, however, I realized that it did not resonate with me. It was no watershed experience, no sudden realization. I didn't own that description of myself, though looking back it was no doubt true. But at that time I was still in a state of denial. I was a big eater and would not have referred to my occasional one-sitting stuffings as bingeing. That's what they were, of course, and I was a compulsive overeater. But merely describing myself that way did not make it real to me.

My other problem, at least with that chapter of Overeaters Anonymous, was that no one appeared to be succeeding. There was no weighing in, no instruction, no training, no discipline. We all just accepted each other the way we were. There were warm, fuzzy, positive things associated with that. We could be ourselves and let our hair down, but rather than seeking change and improvement, I think we felt we could fail and that our friends at OA would understand. It didn't work for me, but I realize fully that it does for some.

Inside another two years I was out of control again, and when our second child, Chad, was born in December of 1977, photos of me with him in our new home show a pretty big dad with a tiny baby.

I should have known better by then—at age twenty-eight —but I was still susceptible to extravagant claims and fad diets. I got sucked into one of the late-night TV commercials for one of those rotation diets where you fast one day and can eat anything you want the next. It was built on the principle that when your stomach shrinks on fast day you will want less the next day. And that if you deprive yourself of nothing on eating day, you'll look forward to it more. Your total calorie intake may be higher than normal when you're eating, but it will be so low when you're not that your overall intake will be less— and isn't that the proven way to lose weight?

No dieting, no exercise, no diaries, no guilt. Fast one day and gorge the next. On fast day they provided a couple of wafers that were actually a cross between giant pills and bars of soap. I sent away for the stuff, had a last supper, and then looked warily at that huge wafer.

You'll find this typically self-sabotaging, but I realized that my last supper had not set me up or psyched me in properly, so I decided that I would start the rotation on eating day, rather than on fasting day. Fair enough. Who cared? I had the sense that I was heavier than I had ever been before, because I was well past the limits of my scale.

The next day at lunch I felt the need to justify to anyone who watched as I gorged on garlic bread, salad with lots of dressing, deep dish pizza, and a hot fudge sundae that I was indeed on a diet. I extolled the virtues and hard-sold the benefits. I ate so much that day that I was sure I could fast the next without a problem.

I enjoyed a huge meal at home and felt my excitement build for the program. I was getting psyched. I treated myself to a midnight snack of lots of ice cream, then set out my wafers and vitamins for the next day.

That day happened to be a Saturday, which may not have been wise, even if this program made sense—which of course it did not. I was miserable from the get-go. I moped about and mourned through breakfast, was irritable and testy. The wafer proved nothing to look forward to and seemed akin to munching on corkboard. The wait till the next day to eat all I wanted seemed interminable.

I forced myself to endure through lunch and the afternoon, even through dinner. By late evening when it was time for bed, I was really down. I began talking about how this would never work, I couldn't handle it, it didn't make sense, I shouldn't have to do anything this drastic, I wanted something to eat, I would gladly sacrifice the investment, I would get on a sensible program like Weight Watchers again, this alone was enough motivation to eat right in the future, blah, blah, blah.

That was the one time when Dianna said, "Do whatever works and makes you happy. This is no way to live—for you or for us."

That was all the permission I needed, and I ate. And the next day I ate. And as I searched for a new local Weight Watchers or Nutri-system or something, I kept eating.

I finally had to be weighed for an insurance physical and learned that I had reached 355 pounds. I was feeling old and as out of shape as I was. My clothes sizes were spiraling up, and I had no idea where I'd stop. Every Sunday night I resolved to start fresh the next day, and every first of the month was a pretty good food day. If the first of the month happened to fall on a Monday, that was a double whammy and I might be motivated for a few days. That was one reason I thought about titling this book *Monday Monday.*

If you have been a lifelong fellow struggler, you know the significance of Mondays, of starting over, of turning over a new leaf, of developing a new resolve. Eventually it makes you feel like a total failure. At one point during this period I was chowing down on a huge lunch—which was my norm after skipping breakfast, and I mentioned something about my frustration over diets. A colleague asked if I had given up. It was asked kindly by someone who cared, so I didn't take offense. It did, however, give me pause.

Had I given up? Had I resigned myself to the fact that I was just a big guy with a predisposition to fat? That some people were destined to be big? Was dieting futile, as everyone—including my doctor—had said? (He encouraged me to lose weight but added that he knew the odds were overwhelmingly against long-term success.)

I responded to my friend that, no, one never gives up. "In the back of my mind there is that thought that I will one day make one more significant run at it." In truth, I was near despair, while every other area of my life was idyllic. I covered the pain with humor and wondered what it would take to finally get me off the dime.

I had missed out on so much. I enjoyed roughhousing with my kids, but I couldn't really play softball or basketball the way I wanted to. Table tennis was about all I could endure, and even then, though I reached tournament level, I was not as mobile as I needed to be and often resorted to trick shots, such as quickly switching paddle hands rather than moving my feet to get to the ball.

It seemed to me I had tried every diet available. Nutri-system was becoming popular, but when I smelled that telltale protein powder odor, I couldn't even try it. It reminded me too much of those dark days on the Last Chance Diet. I walked past the lunchroom once when someone was mixing a vanilla packet (it happened to be a normal-sized person, of all things!) and I could smell that stuff from the hall. It nearly made me sick.

Much of my heavy eating was done in private, so people were surprised that I was as big as I was. I had learned to eat large amounts in public without it showing. Butter, dressing, gravy added to the bulk, but that's what everyone else was eating too. I had more rolls and butter than most people, and I also had crackers and cheese. I knew how to finish off a roll or two and take another while people's attention was elsewhere.

At home I didn't have to worry about that. I ate what I wanted when I wanted it.

I was unhealthy, and I knew it. One night I had gone a few hours without eating after a typically big day of eating. Normally, a few hours without eating would justify something to enjoy, maybe some ice cream. We had some of my favorite, and yet I had a feeling I shouldn't eat anything sweet.

That was a strange feeling. I had never been afraid of any kind of food before. I went to bed satisfied but not as full as usual. I had passed up the temptation for ice cream—a first in months. What was wrong with me? Did I have some premonition that sugar was becoming a problem for me, on top of everything else? It was one thing to overeat, it was quite another to poison oneself.

I was ready for a self-cure, another run at it, as I had come to call it. There would be no weighing in, no classes, no announcements. But I didn't want to go blind or develop other diabetes-related maladies, and with my family history I knew that was inevitable.

So I had a plan.

13

Another Run at It

I awoke the next morning feeling better than I had in a long time, and I came to a decision. Sugar was what was killing me. Regardless what else I did in the way of eating, I needed to swear off refined sugar. I knew there was sugar in most every food, but I didn't worry about it in things like catsup or other basically nonsweet foods.

I eliminated from my diet regular pop, candy, cake, cookies, chocolate syrup, pie, pudding—basically all desserts. And what benefits I received! People were impressed by my discipline. They apologized for partaking themselves. I felt much, much better, avoiding the sugar highs and lows, the fatigue. I felt more energetic, and I saw a slight decrease in my weight and the stuffed feeling.

Once again, I was perfectionistic about it. I went without obvious, refined sugar in dessert form for nine full months. I combined that with my new aversion to between meal snacks, and I believe I was healthier. Not healthy. I was still grossly overweight and a compulsive overeater—though I would not yet have described myself that way—but I was certainly in better shape than I would have been had I also allowed myself sugar.

What I did wrong, of course, was to ignore all the other horrible things I was doing to my body with food. I still skipped breakfast, and I had gigantic lunches. I ate out nearly every day, and if it wasn't lots of Mexican food, it was a big burger and a gyros (a Greek pita sandwich) and large fries. On alternate days, I indulged in my favorite deep dish pizza and garlic bread.

Kidding myself, I believed that being off sugar justified my eating virtually anything else I wanted. I was not attuned to the dangers of fatty foods, and when I put my current, calorie-counting computer program to those days of prodigious eating, I find that I was not terribly far from the calorie totals and fat percentages during my darkest period as a twenty-year-old.

It wasn't unusual for me to start the day with a salad and five tablespoons of creamy garlic dressing, then get another five tablespoons of that dressing, into which I dipped a full order of garlic bread. I think I craved the salt, the fat, and the taste, but, no doubt, there was also sugar in that dressing. I agree that was a pretty bizarre appetizer for half a large, deep dish Chicago-style pizza. So, after skipping breakfast, I got my culinary day started with a lunch totaling 3,150 calories, of which 41 percent came from fat.

On days when I began with a gyros sandwich, a third-pound cheeseburger, and large fries, I was consuming 2,640 calories at 57 percent fat—for lunch alone. As I've said, I rarely eat that much in a whole day now, and never with those fat percentages. Yet by avoiding sugar and having a normal-to-large, standard, home-cooked dinner every night and snacking only on fruit, I thought I was doing fairly well.

I do recall when I first fell off the nonsugar wagon. I was on a business trip to San Francisco and had enjoyed a big, Oriental lunch. My host then served a plate of what appeared to be salted crackers. Wrong. They were wafers filled with the famous Ghiardelli's chocolate. I popped one of those babies in my mouth, and it exploded with luscious flavor. I must have appeared like an alcoholic getting a surprise drink. I downed several of those cookies and—irrational as are most compulsive overeaters—found myself justifying a large hot fudge sundae after dinner that night.

I was off the wagon for a week or so until I began feeling the heart palpitations, the highs and lows, and the aches and pains upon waking. I also saw myself bloating, and so I indulged in a sort of sugary last supper—with ice cream and chocolate candies—and went back to my high-calorie, high-fat, high-sodium, no-snacking, two-gigantic-meals-a-day killer of a program.

Ironically, my weight had gone up to around 360 and stayed there. I somehow had learned to maintain that weight with a 4,000-plus calories per day diet and very little activity, let alone exercise. When I ate more than was even normal for someone my size, I tended to compensate the next few days and stayed even. My joke at that time was, "When I overeat one day, I fast the next. Right now I owe myself seven years."

My waist was about 57 inches, though I never bought pants with a waist larger than 54. I wore size 60 suits and jackets. My shirts were 4-XLs, though I could have gotten by with 3-XLs. I had learned to dress comfortably and camouflage the full extent of my bulk. No one would have guessed me at over 350, but few would have guessed me under 300. People were always surprised to see how tall I was in pictures. In person, my width made me look shorter.

---

*I had everything in
the world to live for:
a great family, many friends,
challenging work, a ministry
—you name it.*

I began falling off the sugarless wagon more and more frequently, and that really took a toll. I would get addicted to chocolates and find myself buying some every day, then buying one last box to signal the end of that. Only the next day I would talk myself into some more. When I added a half pound of chocolate-covered almonds (1,272 calories at 66 percent fat) to my already high-fat diet, I was in mortal danger.

Meanwhile, I had been seemingly happy and productive for years. Michael, our third son, was born in 1982. We had moved to a bigger place on several acres. I had written dozens of books and become vice president for publishing at Moody. I had everything in the world to live for: a great family, many friends, challenging work, a ministry—you name it. I had convinced myself that basically my weight was a given, my eating habits set. Being generally off sugar was keeping me as healthy as possible, and, though I missed out on a lot of physical activity, the fun I couldn't remember from earlier, more mobile days wouldn't hurt me. It was still fun to impress people with how agile I could be at table tennis or how much endurance I had walking through airports. One colleague said he expected me to whine and stop to rest every few hundred feet like his other fat friend.

But when my secretary lost more than ninety pounds, I was inspired anew. I had found myself more and more into sugar and my weight harder to keep steady. She began working at a diet center, and so I decided to go there with my wife— after a last supper on Dianna's birthday—and weigh in. I had been listening to tapes on the neuropsychology of weight control, which called for a lot of visualizing of yourself as a trim and healthy and active person and then eating all you wanted of low-fat foods.

I'm not doing justice to the fundamentally sound program, but, basically, nothing was prohibited while fats were carefully counted. You could enjoy plenty of what you could have. No starving, no serious deprivation. This program encouraged some daily form of exercise. I chose walking.

I took several days to get used to the idea and continued to listen to the tapes and plan. I was a little afraid of the visualizing stuff, having a natural prejudice against anything that sounded New Age. But there was nothing wrong with imagining myself as a different body type.

During the psyche-up period I was at a convention and had breakfast with publisher friends. I noticed that they ate things such as yogurt and granola and fruit. I had hash browns and gravy, sausages, eggs, toast with butter—everything that wasn't good for me. When I talked about my upcoming program, one of my friends pointed to my plate and said, "I used to eat like that. Heart couldn't take it."

He was not being unkind, merely factual. I had hardly thought about what I had chosen for breakfast. I rarely ate breakfast, but when out like this and at an appointment, I ate socially. Something else that was hard for me to imagine: ever passing up such tasty choices. That seemed so foreign to me that I could hardly fathom it.

I told myself, and Dianna, that this would be a birthday present to her. She had neither demanded nor asked, and she was fairly neutral in her response. She was glad I was eager to get going again, but she wanted to make clear that she would support me either way. I really wanted to honor how she had accepted me and stood behind me through years of frustration and failure. And yet we both knew I had to do this for *me*, with motivation from within.

This was the program that really showed me the folly of my perfectionism. Again, like any other diet rooted in calorie and fat percentages, consuming fewer calories than you burn, changing your lifestyle, and eating real, natural foods, there was nothing at all wrong with the idea. It would work if I stayed with it.

I weighed 362.5 on November 13, 1988, and I even had a couple of Polaroid pictures taken. The next day I walked a mile, slowly and carefully, in the frigid weather, ate the natural, low-fat foods they recommended, missed some of the good things I had enjoyed, and almost immediately began feeling great. I enjoyed being hungry again, but I was sore from walking. I found it boring and lonely, so I began taking my almost-eleven-year-old Chad with me.

He was great because he asked typical kid questions. "If the Milky Way fell on Waverly Street, would it hit our house?" I think so.

That was a great time for us, and I was absolutely committed to walk every day, working up to an hour at a time. A clear memory for me was wearing a lined trench coat the first several weeks and not being able to see my feet as we walked.

107

The more we walked and the better I did on the program —only occasionally scooping a spoonful or two of scalloped potatoes out of the serving dish—the more I noticed that on the road I could see the tips of my toes peeking out from under my belly. That was progress. I also noticed that my walking course seemed to shrink. What seemed a long way a few weeks before was now manageable. I flew past my earlier stopping points just barely warmed up.

My weight began to drop slowly and steadily, and I had the idea that I had finally found a sensible program. I was thirty-nine years old, however, and I was also aware of my age catching up with me and fighting this weight loss effort.

Day after day after day Chad and I walked. If I was traveling, I walked in whatever city I found myself. If I had to work late and Chad was already in bed, I would walk alone at midnight. A perfectionist, I would never miss. I had shinsplints, sore ankles and knees, and never looked forward to the walk except for the time I could spend with Chad, but still I kept walking.

I had the very real sense that if I ever strayed from my absolute commitment to walking every day, my resolve would waver, I would begin walking less and less and eventually fizzle out. That was a self-actualizing prophecy, of course. It didn't have to be. But I knew that would be the result. And so I was committed.

As fall gave way to winter, I walked in the snow. I used aerobic tapes and walking tapes to keep me on track and on pace. I kept track of my heart rate, and I was encouraged when I seemed to grow stronger and felt less pain. I could see almost my entire foot with each stride now. My waist was shrinking, the pounds were shedding, and people noticed.

I landed a major book contract and eagerly pursued it. When I was in California, interviewing all day, I walked in the wee hours of the night and tried to be selective about my food. When writing in Chicago in January, having to stay downtown for several days, the only time I could walk was after midnight—alone on scary, frigid streets. I did it.

I once walked fifteen minutes in a blizzard before being forced to turn back, my eyes stinging and my face nearly frozen. But at least I had walked.

One day, a typically crass colleague said to my secretary on the elevator, in front of me, "Don't put your weight back on, now—like he always does." I didn't smile. Neither did she.

I stayed at it and enjoyed the attention. I recall doing well with the food selections and staying on that program fairly well. I was becoming more and more worried about the walking, however. It became less and less appealing and attractive to me, but I was scared to scale back because I just knew I would eventually give it up.

I don't recall why I missed my daily walk on the seventy-eighth day of my program. All I know is that I tried to get right back to it the next day. I did, and I noticed no difference in my rate of weight loss. But just as I had predicted, I missed another day the next week. Then two the following week. Then three.

I was desperate, feeling like a failure, trying to stay with the eating program while the exercise was waning. They began to play on each other. I told myself I could cut my intake even more and quit worrying about the walking. Eventually, of course, because I couldn't handle my commitment having withered, both areas of the program fell by the wayside. I gained my weight back so quickly it was frightening.

I bloated and ballooned. Seemingly overnight I was right back to my largest clothes and my old eating habits. Lost fat and muscle both come back as fat, and they come back fast. After having lost about forty pounds, I rocketed back up and over the 360 mark. The picture on the back of this book was taken in June the following year, 1989, just a few months after I had gained back my forty-pound loss and added at least another fifteen. My guess is that I now weighed in the vicinity of 375 pounds.

For the first time, I really felt my age and my weight. As you can see, there was no hiding it now. I was more than just big. I was fat. I was bloated. I was stuffed. I couldn't imagine room for any more pounds, and yet they just kept coming.

14

Nearing the End of My Rope

I can't emphasize enough how private was this battle. I never admitted to anyone, other than the occasional fellow struggler, any frustration or desperation. My life was otherwise rich and full and happy, and in front of people I always watched what I ate. No desserts in public. Careful maneuvering not to appear to be eating so many rolls or sticky buns or whatever.

I treated my weight, and all of life, with the humor it deserved. "I'm not taking this seriously, so don't you either." I was now in full bloom with my fat humor, and everywhere I spoke, I started with that. Sometimes I was asked to do only comedy, and often fat humor was all I used. Most people loved it. Wasn't it great that this big fat guy could have himself in such healthy perspective?

I really felt I did. Except that I was not feeling well. It had been so long since I felt good that I hardly knew the difference. I was used to being out of breath. I was used to sleeping like a log and having trouble getting out of bed. I was used to always being warm, even in the dead of winter. I didn't own a sweater. I hardly ever wore, let alone buttoned, a coat. I never wore a sports jacket in a car, and rarely indoors. I didn't own a long-sleeved shirt. I never expected to get more than one day's wear out of anything but the occasional pair of pants.

I called airlines early and often to be sure of an aisle seat. But I couldn't have the armrest down. Tray tables stayed up as I held food trays in my lap. I needed a seat-belt extender.

I stood in line at an amusement park for two hours to ride on the big roller coaster only to find that I was unable to fit in the car when it was my turn.

Getting into and out of my own car was an ordeal.

When in a group setting, I had learned to pull my chair away from others in the row so that people would have room to sit next to me.

I looked for places to sit in rooms that had theater-style seating, because there were always spots where extra space had to be left to make the configuration work.

At a board meeting I once slouched too far forward on a metal chair and it gave way, leaving a rear-end shaped scoop in the seat, effectively destroying it. I recall the others being very good about it and not making a joke. They were relieved when I made light of it. I asked if I could take it home and have it mounted. You can imagine the humiliation.

Once, in a meeting at a client's office, I found myself in one of those metal molded chairs that have no back legs. When I sat back in it, the thing began to fold down on itself, so I had to sit forward the whole time. Otherwise, it would have gradually sunk to the floor.

Worst of all was being at an official function where we quasi dignitaries sat in plastic folding chairs outdoors on a gravel-covered lot during a half-hour ceremony. I was in the middle and thus could not make extra space by moving my chair without making a scene. So I turned sideways, squeezed in as carefully as possible, and began to settle in. But my chair, which was not up to someone of my bulk, began to strain against the ground as soon as I sat down. It felt for all the world as if it would go flat in front of hundreds of people. I didn't dare put all my weight on it.

I had to pretend to be sitting when in truth I was just squatting—my seat on the chair but my weight on my thighs and calves. I had no choice. It may sound funny now, but it was one of the most excruciating times of my life. During the prayer I actually stood to get a breather, then squatted again as the prayer neared its end. By the conclusion of the ceremony, my face was beet red, I was sweating profusely, and my legs were cramped and shaking from the exertion.

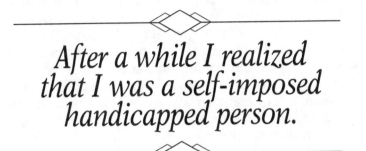

After a while I realized that I was a self-imposed handicapped person.

I would walk two hundred feet out of the way to avoid taking a six-step flight of stairs. If I had no choice but to walk up a couple of flights, I had to rest in the middle or wait at the top and spend several minutes catching my breath before making my entrance.

When walking with a colleague, I could keep up and was proud of it. But don't ask me to also speak. I huffed and puffed and didn't want anyone to know it, so if I was forced to answer a question I would build in dramatic pauses and flourishes to make it sound natural.

After a while I realized that I was a self-imposed handicapped person. I deeply resented people who implied that fat people were merely lazy or undisciplined, though that was exactly how I saw myself. Life wasn't fair. I knew of people who ate a lot and never gained. And yet I could never claim that I wasn't a big eater. Other people claimed it for me, and I didn't argue. But I knew the truth. For whatever reason, I was an overeater, and I wasn't getting better.

With my family history I knew I was a walking time bomb for blood sugar. I'd had bouts with gout, heart palpitations, backaches, and headaches. I was fortunate to have had only marginally high blood pressure, no cholesterol problems, and no depression. I was a very even, usually upbeat person without a temper, generally not argumentative, and known as a fun guy to be with in public and private.

My life was wonderful, except for my private hell.

How long can I go on like this? I wondered. When would heart disease or diabetes or gall bladder problems strike? Had I merely been lucky so far? I conserved energy, moved little. That only contributed to my problem, of course. People didn't even ask me to help lift or carry things. I was treated the way you would treat an old person or someone in a wheelchair. I could tell myself that people were deferring to me for some other reason, but in reality it was because I was unhealthy and it showed.

One summer day I noticed strange patterns in the vision of one eye. I had never suffered that before, but there was no pain. I didn't have a clue that it should mean anything, and when it passed after a while I forgot about it. I was lucky. The pressure behind my eyes was trying to tell me something, but I didn't know enough to have any idea what it might mean.

In the fall of 1990 I noticed that I couldn't seem to change my eye prescription fast enough to keep up with my changing vision. I didn't need bifocals yet, but I was sure having trouble adjusting to the focal differences between things close and far away. I focused easily on a friend at the airport, but when I looked at a clock twenty feet away I had to wait for my eyes to make the adjustment. That was something new. I attributed it to age. I know better now.

Dianna and I took an international trip that fall, and—as usual—I lost weight on the journey. I am always careful what I eat overseas, and we happened to be in the Eastern bloc where American-style foods were hard to get. Of course, my goal was keep off the fifteen or so pounds I dropped in almost as many days, but I had had such goals before.

When we got back to the States I enjoyed a little more mobility but also began to notice that I was hungrier and thirstier than ever. I had probably put back three or four pounds on the flight home alone, due to finally getting what I considered real food and soft drinks.

I was unable to keep from eating in the States, and yet my weight didn't jump back up as it used to. I found that interesting and encouraging, but also puzzling. It was another clue, but I missed it.

In early 1991 I was asked do my shtick at a meeting in Chicago, where Bill Hybels would later bring a message. I had once worked on a book with Bill, pastor of the famed Willowcreek Community Church. He had encouraged me in past weight loss efforts, kindly encouraging me by saying he'd like me to stay around and that I was needed in the kingdom.

He's a great speaker in tremendous demand, of course, so I made a joke about him during my monologue. I said, "I think it was great of this organization, when they couldn't land a big name speaker, to give a local pastor a chance."

The people enjoyed that, and I got a grin from Bill too. But the rest of my humor was all fat related. It seemed to be going over well with everyone *except* Bill. Afterward people asked if my stuff was on tape.

That was gratifying, but I was eager to get to Bill and tell him how much his message had meant to me. He was talking with several others when I approached, and I was flattered when he took my arm and drew me close while he continued speaking with them. Eventually I realized that he was not just trying to show familiarity or friendship. He had something he wanted to say, and he didn't want me to slip away while he finished with the others.

When they finally dissipated I told him how blessed I'd been by his message. He looked me in the eye and in his direct and loving way—as he, among only a few, can do without offense—said, "And you were funny as usual. But it hurts me when you do that to yourself."

I started to say I was only trying to put people at ease, but he continued. "You know, we need you and your family needs you. I want to see you around and productive a long time."

"Thanks," I said.

"I'm serious. You know, the time is going to come when you may have to do something drastic about your problem."

That was a new way to put it. I sensed he was concerned that he not go too far and offend, so he changed the subject and we parted with pleasantries. But his words, and especially his concern, stayed with me: ". . . you may have to do something drastic about your problem."

Almost imperceptibly over the course of the next several months I began losing weight. I noticed that my clothes fit better, then looser. I felt trim, though I was still well over 350. Any time you're losing, you look and feel better than you do at the same weight on your way up.

I didn't even tell Dianna of this strange phenomenon. I wish I could say it was something I was doing subconsciously as a result of Bill Hybels's exhortation. But it wasn't. If anything, I was eating more than ever, consuming more water and diet pop, eating more sugar, and still losing weight. When I began to suffer from insatiable thirst and frequent elimination, I suddenly realized what was going on. I didn't know much about diabetes, but I knew those were two clear symptoms.

Yet I felt wonderful. Who wouldn't feel great about losing weight steadily, if not quickly, while still eating whatever you wanted? I saw more definition in my face and felt lighter and generally more healthy. But I also knew this was too good to be true, and I told Dianna rather matter-of-factly, "Well, it's finally caught up with me. I'm sure I'm diabetic."

Though I like to be widely read and informed, she naturally doubted that I knew what I was talking about or that I could diagnose myself. She was hoping, of course, that I was wrong. High blood sugar and adult-onset diabetes is more than a nuisance. It's a dangerous condition that can cause arthritis, heart problems, circulatory ailments, glaucoma, and even death. Untreated it leads to gangrene, amputations, blindness, rheumatoid arthritis, and hardening of the arteries.

I checked out several books from the library, and they convinced me I was right. Call it pride, stupidity, or simple procrastination, but I put off calling the doctor. I wanted to proceed in blissful ignorance (at least pretended ignorance), so I could enjoy my usual diet while wasting away. The trouble was, this would mean literal wasting away. I couldn't go on too long, or I would be in deep, irreversible trouble.

The books told me that adult-onset diabetes is common among the morbidly obese at my age. The eye troubles, the thirst, the frequent urination were telltale signs. I kept a close watch on my weight. My scales went up to only 350, so I hadn't been on them in months. Now I noticed that though I was still

116

over the scale limit, the balance was struggling to level itself. That meant I was in the 355 range. A few weeks later I slipped into the 340s. I hadn't been that light, if you can call it that, since my weight loss attempt of nearly two years before.

When I got to the low 340s, I could delay no longer. It was one thing to be losing weight. It was quite another to be testing fate. I was diabetic and I knew it, and I would be the biggest fool of all to pretend otherwise and blithely go on my way, threatening my health and my future when I had a young family. The bottom line was that I had been irresponsible long enough.

It wasn't that I hadn't tried to lose weight. I may have even forgotten some of the diets and plans I tried over the years. If you're a fellow struggler, I'm sure your history is much the same as mine, and that's why I have risked your patience by recounting it. Nearly everyone I know with a significant weight problem has tried all the things I've tried. I know there's more to success that just determination and self-control, and I know there are myriad things working against us.

But now I had to get to the doctor and find out how deeply ingrained was my blood sugar disease and what I would have to do about it. I did not want to be insulin-dependent, certainly not with shots, and I wanted even to avoid oral insulin if I could. The books all talked about controlling diabetes with diet and exercise, and, to tell you the truth, both those words hit me like cold water in the face.

If there was anything that sounded less attractive than watching your weight, watching what you ate, and exercising regularly, it was giving yourself a shot or two of insulin every day. Some people control their diabetes that way and their weight continues to be a problem. If they want to eat more sugar, they simply increase their insulin dose. I never wanted to get into that.

Yet reading about target heart rates and working out was so foreign and so repulsive to me that I began thinking about losing enough weight to get where I could involve myself in some competitive sport. Was I too old? Had I waited too long? Surely I had, but there was no more putting off doing whatever I had to do. I called the doctor.

"I need to come in for a blood test," I said. "I'm sure I'm diabetic."

He told me in essence that he would be the judge of that, but when I told him my symptoms he added, "You're probably right."

The doctor called me when the blood tests came back. "Why don't you come in for a chat?"

15

Something Drastic

I was right, the doctor told me. I was diabetic. My glucose level was 286 on June 5, 1991. My weight had dropped to 338 pounds, but it was not a healthy loss. My cholesterol was not a problem, registering 195, well within the safe zone, especially for someone my size. That was as high as it had ever been. I had always been fortunate with cholesterol and blood pressure.

I was not so fortunate, however, in the area of triglycerides—the true fats in the blood. A normal level of triglycerides is between 50 and 250 milligrams per tenth of a liter of blood. The computer readout registered a maximum of only three digits. No one wanted to guess how much higher my count was than the 999 spit out by the printer.

I claim no scientific or medical knowledge and promise not to allow this book to become complex. Suffice to say, it makes little difference how healthy your cholesterol level appears if your triglycerides are off the charts. I had been reading my books about diabetes and was sufficiently sobered about its severity. I dreaded the idea of a restricted diet and—ugh!—regular exercise, but I was fully prepared for some hard advice from the doctor.

He told me that we had diagnosed the diabetes early enough that it had done no permanent damage. The good news was that my pancreas was producing insulin, just not enough for someone my size. The doctor put me on a low oral dose of insulin until I got into a weight loss program. His recommendation was that I lose a hundred pounds and keep it off. He said this knowing it would come as no surprise to me, and he also said he knew that the long-term potential of success was minuscule. The other option? More insulin orally until it became necessary to take it by injection. In essence, he added, that was no way to live, and, if I was counteracting obesity and blood sugar through medication, I would not be much healthier than I was now.

I was not yet psyched or sure that I was ready for yet another run at significant weight loss. By now you are as bored with my efforts as I was in making them. If I hadn't tried *everything*, I had tried a derivative of everything. The only light at the end of my tunnel was that I had never resorted to blaming the particular program. The programs had not failed. I had. Unless a diet claimed it could overcome human weakness, it never promised more than it could deliver if I did my part.

I could not let diabetes have its way with my body without fighting it with all that was in me.

I am grateful that my doctor was realistic, because he would not have been able to scare me, shock me, or Dutch uncle me into being motivated. Nearly my entire adult life has been dedicated to my family. I don't merely write and speak about family priorities; I am obnoxious about them. I set and maintain personal policies that give me megablocks of time with my wife and kids. At the time of my diagnosis my wife was in her early forties and my boys were fifteen, thirteen, and nine. I was forty-one. I had all the motivation I needed.

I hinted earlier that uglier parts of my story were forthcoming, and we have come to one of those places. The following paragraphs are ones I would just as soon gloss over or skip entirely, but when I decided to tell this story I committed to telling it all.

The hardest part of my conclusions will come later, when I finally get a tenuous handle on the whys—the psychological reasons for my compulsions. But here I must explain another unpleasant truth I have learned about myself, something I knew subconsciously all along but that came raging to the fore when I was diagnosed with diabetes and informed that the only viable, potentially long-term successful approach was to lose my excess weight and keep it off. That, of course, meant the clichéd "change of lifestyle," "change of eating habits," etc., etc.

To cut to the chase, let me begin by saying that I realized immediately that I had no choice. For all that I had ever said about outside motivation, this was something that could not be ignored. I could not let diabetes have its way with my body without fighting it with all that was in me. For the sake of my family? You bet. And that meant for my sake as well.

As a Christian, how could I do otherwise? And yet, had I not been a Christian nearly all my life? Had I not known my body was the temple of the Holy Spirit who lives in me? What would make me any more devout or committed or successful this time? A little more outside motivation? The guilt of leaving my family husbandless, fatherless?

These were the things I had to think through, because something was playing at the edges of my brain, and it was something I didn't like, something I didn't want to deal with. For one thing, I knew I was going to do this. I was going to get myself psyched, do this thing right—once and for all—and wage a never-ending battle for the rest of my life.

But what was that ugliness that threatened to creep in on me? It was this: I knew beyond doubt that, left to my own devices, I would rather eat the way I wanted to, be unhealthy, and die—were it not for my family.

Now maybe that was a big buildup for a big letdown. Maybe you were expecting that some memory of childhood abuse came rushing to my mind. No. What came to me was the realization that I was no better than an alcoholic or a drug addict who would sacrifice everything dear to him for his addiction. I hated psycho-babble. I hated the term *eating disorder.*

But when I saw specials about young drug addicts who go into recovery, I saw myself. They spend the first few days in denial, telling the newly recovered addicts that they themselves were not addicted, that they could quit at any time. It takes someone else, someone who has been through the program, to challenge them, to tell them, "You love your drugs more than you love your family, your parents, your brothers and sisters, your wife, your kids."

The newcomer gets mad and argues and fights. He resists and resists until his craving for drugs gets so strong that he realizes, yes, he would trade his baby for a hit.

Too severe a comparison? Need I really put myself in that category? Only if I decided not to lose the weight and keep it off.

It was no easy, flippant decision. As I've said, I really had no choice, but what would my preference have been? To my shame, especially as a Christian, I reiterate: Were it not for my family, I would choose to eat the way I want.

It's not difficult to see why that is so ugly and why I would just as soon not admit it. In Philippians 3:18–19, Paul writes of many "of whom I have told you often, and now tell you even weeping, that they are the enemies of the cross of Christ: whose end is destruction, whose god is their belly, and whose glory is in their shame—who set their mind on earthly things." I'm not enough of a theologian or scholar to know why enemies of the cross, whose end is destruction, whose glory is in their shame, and who set their mind on earthly things are in the same list as those whose god is their belly. But there it is.

Besides the painful mirror that Scripture provides, something else was playing at my mind. It shouldn't surprise you that by this time in my life, with everything else seemingly under control, the last thing I needed was another dieting failure. This time a failure would result in battling diabetes with external insulin. But even aside from the medical dangers, I was the classical yo-yo dieter who had proved he could not maintain a weight loss.

The combination of knowing I had no choice and yet facing the truth about myself contributed to an unusual resolve. On the one hand, I resented that my choice was really *no* choice. On the other, as long as I had to do this anyway, somehow, some way, I had to do it right.

It would have been easier, I think (and as I said earlier), to have found some psychological reason for my problem. I took no comfort in the fact that my failure was in good, broad company. I wanted to, needed to—simply had to—succeed this time, regardless of my history or that of anyone else.

I began hearing the statistics. Some said only 1 in 1,000 people who take off more than a hundred pounds keep it off for more than a year. And a full 50 percent of the rest gain back more than they lost.

I had to forget statistics. I even had to ignore my doctor's realism, which to a struggler appeared fatalistic. It was as if he were saying, "You must try this even if it doesn't work."

An early and positive conclusion I reached was that one of the problems I might have had in the past was that I *did* have a choice. Of course I had wanted to lose weight and keep it off, but I hadn't wanted that as badly as I wanted to eat the way I wished.

For a few days, as I pondered this no-choice choice, I thought a lot about how committed, determined, obsessive, uncompromising, and sold-out I would have to be to make this work. I needed no other horror stories to scare me. My personal history was my own worst enemy. I had as bad a track record as any dieter I could think of, and, like anyone else, I knew hardly anyone who had maintained a significant weight loss.

My doctor suggested a new program at Victory Memorial Hospital in nearby Waukegan, Illinois, called New Direction. It had been developed by Ross Laboratories, a division of Abbott Laboratories, a leading pharmaceutical company headquartered not far from us. He gave me the name of the program director at Victory, Bruce Yamamoto.

Our first meeting was by phone. Bruce, an earnest, soft-spoken man in his mid-thirties, explained that New Direction was basically a fast, supplemented by all-liquid protein, diet Jell-O, and caffeine-free diet pop. Before I could back out, based on my experience nearly fifteen years before on the so-called Last Chance Diet, he explained how far technology, medical monitoring, and research had come in the years since such diets were considered dangerous. I was still listening.

He also explained that the program wasn't for everyone. There was extensive initial screening, blood work, and even an interview with a behaviorist. There was little doubt in my mind that I would qualify, and I even began thinking about how well I would do. Also, Bruce said, the program was not cheap. On the other hand, the cost wouldn't be much different from what I would pay for the large amount of food I would otherwise consume during the same period.

Slowly I became excited about the possibilities, but I retained a careful wariness. What if I didn't like the beverage? What if I couldn't stand the protein powder smell? What if the behaviorist was a New Age weirdo who thought I needed a shrink?

My first visit to Victory Memorial is etched in my memory. I recall parking and slowly strolling in, noticing the beautifully kept, gleaming facility. I loved the name. Victory. That was what I needed over the one area in my life where I had always ultimately failed.

I met with Bruce—who appeared about the total weight that I needed to lose. He explained that New Direction was a program with medically monitored rapid weight loss and group classes where we would study behavior modification, nutrition, and exercise. I ignored the third, because it loomed as a mountain I didn't want to think about. Anyway, I knew I was too big, too out of shape, and too unhealthy to start exercising yet. Besides, they didn't recommend it during the initial stages of the program.

He described the three phases of the program: *reducing* (on a very low calorie diet—or modified fast—for as long as it takes to reach your goal), *adapting* (a five-week period where food is reintroduced), and *sustaining* (six months).

Bruce had me sample the powder, which was to be mixed with water three times a day (in my case, four—which is true of most men and unusually large women). The program was designed only for people significantly overweight.

The beverage came in chocolate, chocolate with fiber, and vanilla (with five different flavor packets to add variety). There was also a chicken soup flavor, which was to be mixed with hot water. Bruce warned me that this last flavor was generally not popular with clients but that those who liked it really liked it.

I found the chocolate palatable and the protein smell mild enough. The vanilla was very bland, but I would try some of the flavor packets. I thought the chicken soup would appeal once I had quit eating and could pretend that it was a heartier meal. (I tried it once. Ugh!)

The different packets were roughly 220 calories each, so I would be consuming 880 calories a day, plus a few in the diet colas and sugar-free Jell-O. Stunning to me was that they could very accurately predict your weight loss by a simple formula. It went like this:

Multiply your current weight by twelve; the total is the average number of calories you need per day to maintain your present weight. Subtract from that the number of calories you will consume per day on the modified fast, and the figure that results is your calorie debt. In other words, at 341 pounds, I would have had to consume roughly 4,092 calories to maintain. That minus 880 was a calorie debt of 3,212. As it takes 3,500 calories to gain or lose a pound, I divided the 3,212 into 3,500 and came up with 1.09, which is the number of days it would take me to lose a pound.

How to Predict Weight Loss

Current weight × 12 = Daily calories needed to maintain weight

Calories needed to maintain – Calories consumed = Calorie debt

3,500 ÷ Calorie debt = No. of days to lose 1 lb.

With that formula, I should have lost about six pounds a week, but of course the formula changes every time a person's weight changes. The prediction was that if I did not cheat and allowed my body to stay in a state of ketosis, I would lose a large amount of water weight the first few weeks and then settle in at about a five-pound per week loss for almost as long as it would take to reach my goal. *Ketosis* was defined as the state in which the body, in effect, burns itself as fuel when all other reserves are gone. The danger is that you lose muscle mass, which must be carefully monitored. The nuisance is that it gives you what the New Direction people called "fruity breath." We clients decided it was three-week-old fruit! Call it trench breath.

So that was the basic program: a modified, all-liquid fast with heavy calorie debt. It was intimidating, daunting, and severe. And I came to believe I was made for it and vice versa.

I then had my appointment with the behaviorist, Sarah Bieber, who was even tinier than Bruce. She was a young, thin blonde with sparkling eyes and a clear concern for her potential patients. I would have been even more encouraged if both Bruce and Sarah had been program success stories with "before" pictures that showed their prodigious girths. But no. As would also be true with the dietician I would meet eventually, the three principal care givers in New Direction were lifelong civilians—very trim, attractive people who proved expert, but not due to personal experience.

The first question Sarah asked me was, "Why do you think you're overweight?"

I suppose I should have tried to determine what she was driving at. Was she asking why I was an overeater, or was she asking if I had a clue that food had something to do with this? I assumed that it was the former, and so I told her what I have told you: "I don't know. I see no psychological reasons for why I should be an overeater."

She was intrigued, or seemed to be, and we had a lengthy, animated conversation that convinced me, above all else, that I would enjoy working with her. She was committed and determined and sympathetic.

Before she asked, I told her that one thing I was tired of was people telling me that I had to learn what made me fat and how to eat right, get thin, stay thin, and all that. "I'm sure there are things I don't know and things it will be very helpful for me to get handles on," I said. "But trust me—no one knows more about what makes a person fat or thin than a fat person."

Sarah had a good sense of humor and, I presume, gave me a relatively clean bill of psychological health.

Somewhere in the midst of all this—the thinking about it, talking about it, praying about it, and worrying about it—I committed myself. And I mean committed. I decided that I would finally do something drastic, that I would be absolutely resolute. I would go on the modified fast for as long as it took to get to my goal, and I would not cheat one bite, not one.

16

Jumping In

I predicted my perfection on the reducing phase to the staff at New Direction, and each cautioned me not to be so dogmatic. They were concerned with my perfectionism and feared that if I cheated once after such a declaration, I might cash in the whole thing the way I had my neuropsychology walking program.

They may have been right, and perfectionism proved to be a hurdle. But there was no doubt in my mind, none, that if I did this, I would do it right.

My blood test results were as bad as they had been before, and I was informed that I would be enduring those every two weeks during the reducing phase because it was dangerous and they wanted to be on top of all changes in my body. I was excited to know that I had been accepted and that I would officially begin June 20, 1991.

By then I would have had many last suppers—which were not recommended by New Direction but reluctantly accepted as normal. Over the few weeks between my initial blood work and my first weigh-in, I gained three pounds and began the New Direction experience at 341. Significantly, though I didn't realize it at the time, my blood pressure was 138/86 and my resting pulse rate 80. That was not atypical for someone my size, but it was not healthy either.

Though I looked ahead with great fear to several weeks on a virtual fast, the promise that I would lose weight quickly appealed to me. I would not have been able to endure some year-long (or longer) restrictive diet that saw me drop two pounds a week or less. I needed and wanted immediate, encouraging results.

By that first day I was as psyched and encouraged a patient as they could ask for. I liked the idea of a weekly class with fellow strugglers, some of whom had begun months before and were losing steadily, some who were cheating and struggling, and a few who were starting the same day I was.

At the beginning the group was composed of mostly middle-aged and older women, a young man, and another guy about my age telling our stories. How long have you been on the program, how much have you lost, and how is it going? A couple of people had been on the program two months and had lost dozens of pounds. They were excited and encouraging. A couple of others were fighting a tendency to cheat.

When it was my turn I said I had been on the program about twenty minutes and that I couldn't wait to see how much I had lost already. I also made the rash-sounding prediction that I would not cheat, not one bite. Everyone looked at me bemused, but that made me only more determined. I knew beyond doubt that I would not cheat, but declaring it like that would also help me when my resolve was weak.

One thing I was completely certain of and decided to tell myself frequently every day was, "This is the easy part." Anybody, especially I, can lose weight. The hard part comes when the losing is over. You don't want to know how many times I told myself that.

Shortly after I began the program, my doctor gave me a treadmill test because of my childhood history of rheumatic fever. He detected some residual damage, but nothing that would restrict my physical activity once I lost enough weight to get into it. He did prescribe half an aspirin a day to keep my blood thin. That remains the only medication I am on today.

I recount my losing experience here only for illustration. Such a weight loss program may not be right for you or appeal to you in the least. But if you want immediate, encouraging results, it just may be. I recommend any doctor-suggested, medically monitored program that is nutritious, sensible, and calls for consuming fewer calories than you burn.

Despite how often I told myself that losing was the easy part, it was not easy. I was so committed and so resolute that I was not even tempted to quit or to cheat, but I endured some bitterly difficult days, especially at first.

Of course, I was reminded of the depression I went through when I had first tried the fasting diet in the mid-1970s. But this was something different. We were advised to drink prodigious amounts of water, and caffeine- and sugar-free beverages as well, which I did with a vengeance. But while experimenting with the packets and the coldness of the water and all that, I was frustrated. If I mixed and drank a concoction I didn't really enjoy, I was disappointed and almost despairing. I drank a protein beverage roughly at the three meal times and then another at 9:00 P.M.

I drank water and other legal beverages in the meantime, trying to stave off the headaches and hunger pangs. They were severe and trying, but they were nothing compared to what I can describe only as grief. I mourned the loss of food, the loss of the fun of eating with my family or out with friends. I missed everything about it, especially the taste. Possibly worst of all was a sense of foreboding, of having nothing to look forward to.

I could hardly believe the number of triggers that reminded me it was nearly mealtime. Then I would realize that I wouldn't be having an actual meal but rather a packet of powder and nine ounces of water. I eventually learned that I did not enjoy any of the flavors except chocolate—and that only with very cold, icy water. This I shook in a special container and drank in one series of gulps. Others told me they nursed their drinks for several minutes. I couldn't. To me, this was medicinal, and I treated it as such. I wasn't really eating; I was taking in just enough fuel to stay alive while I dealt with my excess weight.

For the first several days I found myself actually weepy, melancholy, sad. In a way that disgusted me. I had joked in the past that all my landmarks were food oriented. "Go to McDonald's. Turn left till you come to Pizza Hut . . ." Now I realized that my life had literally revolved around meals. I planned my day by them, looked forward to them, and despaired when I could not have them.

As I looked ahead I saw days, weeks, months of the same, and I was nearly overcome. As I've said, I was not tempted to give in, and I wasn't about to cheat. Even though a cracker or a cookie or a chip here and there would not have made that much difference, the only way to get the most out of the program was to stick with it, do it right, and stay in ketosis. Any little bite had the potential of slowing down ketosis and prolonging the fast. I don't know why they call it a fast when it goes so slow!

After a few days, the headaches and hunger disappeared, and they were gone for good. Physically I began to feel marvelous. I could feel the pounds melting away. I was proud of myself and knew this was going to work, but I was still mourning. There was absolutely no physical hunger. This is largely true with New Direction patients, though I know a few who said they were hungry the whole time.

I was aware of mental and mouth hunger. I was jealous of people who could eat, and I resented that I could not. I blamed myself, of course. It was I who had gotten myself into this state.

Again I became aware of the array of food triggers out there. Commercials, conversations, signs, logos, smells, colors, locations, everything. The trip home from the class at the hospital every week reminded me of great Mexican restaurants, ice cream places, fast-food joints, pizza, candy bars, and cookies at the gas station. It was torture, but it was all in the mind. I was so grateful that the physical hunger had disappeared! I'm not saying I didn't want to eat. Just that the lack of hunger made it possible for me not to cheat.

At the end of the first week I couldn't wait to weigh in and see how I had done. I wanted to see everyone again and talk to the dietician, Sue Jeep. She was closer to my age, but like Sarah she was small and thin. What was it with these people? I still think Bruce, Sarah, and Sue should have found people with similar color and features and bought their fat pictures. Then they could say, "See what the program has meant to us?"

Dark-haired Sue took personal interest and was of tremendous encouragement. I always loved to hear her share the floor with Sarah, covering important dietetic and nutritional information but also showing that concern and compassion that made us all want to succeed.

It was she who helped us set our goals. Mine was set, for the first time realistically, at 240. The charts might have said that I should weigh 194, but how practical was that? Sue assured me that setting an unrealistic goal could be as damaging as never trying.

What a thrill it was to weigh in at 327 at the end of that first week. My blood pressure was at a more normal 124/80, and my resting pulse was already down to 72. Most incredible, my glucose level dropped from 286 to 107 in 21 days! My uric acid was up, and I began feeling the twinges of gout, but a quick prescription nipped that.

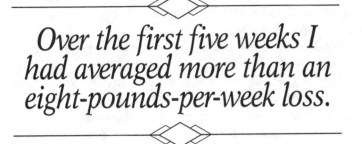

Over the first five weeks I had averaged more than an eight-pounds-per-week loss.

I was so encouraged by the results and by what we were talking about in class that I knew I could carry on despite the fact that we skipped the next week due to the Fourth of July. My goal was to lose another thirteen pounds over the next two weeks, and I hit that right on the nose. I was on vacation the next two weeks, but I was rigid and successful again and dropped fifteen pounds.

I had lost forty-two pounds in five weeks, and I was dropping so fast they considered adding a packet of beverage to my daily intake. They didn't want me losing too much muscle mass. I was thrilled and felt as if I would soon level off to a more realistic weekly figure.

I was obsessed with the program, with the fast, with food, with talking about it. I'm sure I drove my family crazy. I began to look forward to my beverages, and when I discovered how good sugar-free Jell-O was, I considered it almost food. I had a cup of it with every beverage and told many people I thought it had saved my life.

I still hated the fact that I didn't have meals to look forward to, but that was getting a little easier too. My blood pressure was down to 114/72, my pulse down to 68, and—best of all—I had slipped under 300 pounds for the first time in years. Over the first five weeks I had averaged more than an eight-pounds-per-week loss.

One of the first things I noticed was how much time I had on my hands. I had spent more time eating and snacking than I ever realized. Now I was looking for places to go, things to do, things to read, things to watch, things to talk about. It was amazing. I have always been described as a prolific writer. But during the fast my writing volume bordered on the ridiculous. What else was there to do?

I continued to spend a lot of time with my family, but I sensed they humored me. Food, the diet, my weight, the calendar were all I could talk about. I was aware of this and knew how annoying it must be, but I could not stop. I would apologize, and they would assure me that it was all right. But a few minutes later I would be talking about it again—something I'd learned or realized, some new vow or pledge, some new appreciation for control or small amounts of food, whatever.

When we were out with others, they were naturally interested in what was happening to me. I couldn't believe my luck: a fresh audience who hadn't heard it all day every day!

Among my goals was to get into decent enough shape to be able to play church softball the next summer. That seemed ages away. I also wanted to be able to cross my legs without holding my breath and hanging onto my ankle with two hands. I even kidded about being able to cross my legs and tuck the crossover toe behind the other calf the way really skinny people do.

As I began to lose, I felt lighter than I was. Even in the high two hundreds, with no protruding stomach, no full feeling, and decidedly smaller than I had been just two weeks before, I moved like a thinner person.

For the next twelve weeks I lost almost exactly five pounds a week every week. I put off buying new clothes and saw everything get baggy. I was energetic, obsessed, obnoxious, and drinking in the praise. My weight plummeted from 299 to 294 to 289 to 284 to 279 to 274 to 269 to 265 to 263 to 254 to 249 to 245 and to 240 on October 17. My resting pulse was down to 60 (normal range is 60–80) and my blood pressure to 110/68.

I had already reached my goal, losing more than 100 pounds in seventeen weeks, but I wasn't finished. I had finally started exercising, trying an exercycle for the first time in years. It took a long time to get used to, and I hated it at first. It didn't take long to get winded and sore, and when I had a smaller than usual weight loss one week, I attributed it to the exercise. I feared I was gaining muscle mass and thus weight, but the following week I lost more than my usual five pounds and was right back on track.

My cholesterol was down into the 140s, and by the time I was finished I would see my triglycerides drop from off the charts at 999 to 104!

Though I had reached my goal, I continued reducing for a few more weeks, waiting for my body to tell me enough was enough. That came when I dropped to 233. Food was reintroduced into my diet slowly, four ounces of protein the first week and other healthy things substituting for one packet per day each week over the next four weeks. By November 28 I had lost even more weight and hit a low of 232—just about the same weight at which I graduated from high school in 1967. It was time for the sustaining phase.

As I had known for weeks, the toughest time was yet to come. That story, and much of what I learned during all those reducing and adapting sessions, I want to share with you in the hope that you can enjoy an adventure similar to mine. Because, as I've said, we all know that there are myriad ways to lose the weight. That has never been the problem. The problem is keeping it off.

17

Lessons from the Trenches

When you're on, up, zoned, psyched, or whatever other cliché fits that feeling of invincibility, you become also ultrasensitive to the baloney factor. I was sailing along, strict on the program, not cheating, losing rapidly, and enjoying my status as the world's largest visual aid.

The rest of the group lovingly hated to hear that I had again gone another week without sneaking a cookie or a piece of fruit. Some would tell of good and bad days, of cheating more or less this week than last. I could always detect rationalization, however, because I had been such a champ at it in the past.

One man, who had begun the program before I did but was approximately my size and losing at my rate, talked about falling off the wagon a couple of times one week. That was one thing. If someone cheated and attributed the lapse to themselves, their own weakness, their own actions, I believed it was healthy. I knew that, though I would likely get through the reducing phase without having faltered, there was no realistic way I would live the rest of my life on some spartan or restricted diet and never have a lapse. I knew reducing was the easy part and that the real battle was yet to come. I wanted to stay attuned to baloney so that I would no longer be able to fool myself.

But this man who had cheated began saying things like, "I was doing well until everybody started telling me that one bite wouldn't hurt, that I should try something. I mean, it was a buffet after all."

As soon as I heard the word *everybody*, I heard rationalization. I was learning to stay away from buffets and from blaming my eating on other people. Perhaps I was bordering on being judgmental, but we all know that we are responsible for what we do. If we cheat, it's because we decide to succumb to outside influences.

I assumed the day would come when I would be looking for reasons why I had lapsed or slipped, and I was determined to keep the blame right where it belonged. While in the reducing phase, I had many people tell me, "You shouldn't starve yourself. One bite won't hurt you. What if you lose your taste for food altogether? I made this just for you. You don't want to offend me, do you?"

My response was, "Why, you sound as if you would offer a drink to an alcoholic!"

They'd laugh and say of course they wouldn't, and I explained that that's how I saw myself currently. "I can enjoy watching others eat, but for now, I can't and I won't."

I must say, some people lost fairly steadily in spite of rather frequent cheating—or what the New Direction staff preferred to call "lapses." Of course, these were discouraged, but the emphasis was on not letting them do you in. I had the very real feeling that if I lapsed, I would fail. And I probably would have, if for no other reason than that I told myself I would.

That perfectionism had long been a problem for me, but not in other areas of my life. Sure, there were things I liked perfect. I enjoy turning out a perfectly spelled and printed page of manuscript. I'm not saying the writing or the content is perfect, but, as it relates to those areas I can control, I want it perfect. If it is not, I fix it and print it out again.

But I'm not a neatnick. I like a clean car, but I can go several days past when it needs a wash without having a personal crisis. I like a neat work area, but when I'm on deadline I can work in the midst of clutter. So I didn't understand my penchant for perfection in following the modified fast or—

worse—in thinking that the only valid exercise program was a religious, daily regimen.

That, I feared, would eventually get me into trouble, and so I began trying to adjust my thinking on it. I was learning from exercise therapists that a good, aerobic program calls for getting your pulse into the target heart rate for at least twenty minutes a day, three days a week. I couldn't imagine being that flexible. In my mind, the only exercise worth doing was something you committed yourself to daily and never missed. But, of course, I had tried that, and the first time I missed, it was virtually over.

Exercise still loomed as a mountain to me. I was thrilled with my rapid weight loss, which at first included no exercise. I was too heavy. My knees hurt. My back ached. I *couldn't* exercise. That was what I thought and said. There was some truth to all that, but the day of reckoning was coming.

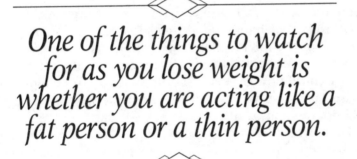

One of the things to watch for as you lose weight is whether you are acting like a fat person or a thin person.

I had spent most of my adult life looking for ways to avoid excess movement. We were taught at New Direction, and I recognized this, that the truly obese person tends to move as little as possible. We don't even move much in our chairs. We settle in and hibernate. We combine trips. If we have to get up to get food or drink or throw something away or find something, we wait until we have accumulated several such tasks, and then we do them all at once. Then we're back, camped out.

Lighter people are more animated. They move around, they gesture more, they move more even in their chairs. They're up, down, they're all around. One of the things to watch for as you lose weight is whether you are acting like a fat person or a thin person.

I mentioned earlier that as I lost quickly, I felt thin. However, in many ways I didn't *act* thin. I continued to find myself sitting still. More revealing, however, was something that made me sympathetic, for the first time, to sufferers of severe eating disorders such as bulimia and anorexia nervosa.

Sad to say, I was insensitive enough in the past to have joked that I wouldn't mind catching a mild case of anorexia. I wouldn't say that in public, of course, but now it is not even the type of thing I would privately kid about. I have learned enough about that horror to no longer find it funny in the least.

I became most sympathetic in this area of body image. When I was huge, pushing 380 pounds, I was unaware how big I looked. No one guessed me that big, so I saw myself (in my mind) as that 275-pound college freshman. Then I would see a picture and be stunned and embarrassed at my mass.

On the other hand, when I was losing, I could not see the difference in the mirror. Every forty pounds or so, New Direction would shoot a Polaroid. In photos, I could see it. In the mirror I could not. Even when I had lost all my weight and—because I was not on food yet—looked actually thin and gaunt at 232 pounds, in the mirror I saw a fat man.

That was shocking to me. Why couldn't I see in real life what I saw in a photograph? People were amazed at the difference in me, especially because I also cut off my years-old beard. Friends I had known forever didn't know me. I said to one woman, "You don't know who you're talking to, do you?"

She said, "No. Who am I talking to?" When I told her she nearly fainted.

People who saw my name under my new picture thought I was dying of cancer. I was pale, frail, had lost muscle mass and tone, and my hair had even thinned and seemed a lighter gray. I was thrilled with my new, lighter feel and my accomplishment, and people complimented me. But I noticed a distinct look of sympathy, shock, and pity in their eyes. I looked like a withered old man. I was assured that my body would return to some sort of tone when I began eating like a normal person. Even at the same weight or ten or fifteen pounds heavier, I would look much different, much healthier—so they said. Of course, I didn't want to put back on even one pound, but I had slid far below my goal, and it wasn't realistic to think I could stay at the same weight I had dropped to on 880 calories a day when I would approximately triple that intake once I was off adapting.

I put the beard back on because I tired of being invisible. I became acutely aware of a difference in how people reacted and responded to me. Once they were used to the new me, they treated me differently than they ever had before. No doubt it was subconscious on both our parts, but I had lost a certain power of presence.

As I said much earlier, I had never been aware of the impact of my size on other people. I didn't feel any different inside and was always surprised to notice in pictures how I dominated a room and was twice the size of most everyone else. But I was not aware what that had meant in interpersonal relationships. Apparently my bulk magnified my every mood, expression, and comment. My humble (or so I thought) opinions were taken as directives. My suggestions seemed like commands. I seriously did not intend this, and they were not expressed that way. But I guess it's like the old joke: Where does a 500-pound gorilla sleep? Anywhere he wants. In other words, if a 350–400 pound guy wonders if anyone else wants to go for pizza, they decide they do.

When I was aware that people seemed to naturally defer to me, even when I didn't care one way or the other, I tried to counteract that. Friends told me that they had felt strangely intimidated at first and realized only after they got to know me that I did not intend that. So I had learned to try to bend over backwards to stay in the background, to let others make decisions, to not give my opinion or preference unless it was important or I felt strongly about it. I didn't want to consciously manipulate.

It was when my size had disappeared that I realized what people had been talking about. You never know what you're missing until it's gone, and my power of presence left me virtually overnight.

141

Since I hadn't cultivated my size for power reasons (at least consciously), it was hard to mourn its disappearance. But I was certainly aware of it. I had trouble keeping people's attention as long as I used to. My suggestions and comments carried no more weight (pun not intended) than anyone else's. Perhaps I thought in the past that I did have the best ideas, was the most profound, the funniest, the most persuasive. Judging from how people now reacted to a weak, thin, frail-looking man who suddenly looked even older than his years, I got a rude awakening. At the risk of overreacting, it appeared to me that perhaps my entire power of presence rested in my size.

I felt invisible. I had disappeared. Dianna noticed that I even sat differently. She said that with my weight on I sat up and looked broad shouldered, despite my girth. Now I seemed to cross my legs (easily, finally), fold my arms, lean forward, and collapse in on myself. While sitting with other people I would notice that I had almost folded myself into a closed ball, observing from a small, almost hidden position. I had to remind myself to sit up straight and hold my chin up.

The irony of all this was that in the 230s I was still one of the heaviest men in any room, unless a really big man arrived. Yet I felt small and weak. My joke became, "I'm finally in shape, and now I'm old."

That had been my reaction when I first shaved my beard. I looked at this pale, skinny face, and the sagging skin at my neck (not so elastic as I had been years before), and I looked more like my father than ever. Though I had always looked older than my years because of graying prematurely, my size had also contributed to that. Now, because my neck was thin and my clothes too big and my muscles too small, I had aged even more. I had no problem resembling my father. That is inevitable, and I could sure do worse. But he is twenty-six years older than I, and I would happily wait many years before looking like I could be his brother.

Believe me, I was glad to be back on food. When we first began hearing about four-ounce servings of chicken or fish and all kinds of fruits and vegetables, I couldn't imagine getting along on that. In the months prior to my diagnosis and recommended treatment, I had become addicted to quarter-pounders with cheese, and I wondered if I would ever be able to shake that.

For weeks on the fast, I dreamt of those burgers. I also had dreams about blowing the program on cakes, pies, ice cream, and cookies, even though a sweet tooth had never been my problem. Sugar was the one area I had usually been able to control. I was learning from the program that my real addiction had been to fat. I looked forward to the day that those burgers I craved would seem like the enemy to me.

That day came late in the fast when those tiny portions we would get during adapting all of a sudden seemed like feasts. What a revelation that was to me, that I could look forward to three ounces of shrimp, four ounces of chicken, two ounces of beef. I knew that wouldn't last; these were simply the types of portions that would be carefully reintroduced during the adapting (to normal food) stage. I began to yearn for that kind of a meal.

I had stayed away from the kitchen during family meals while on the beverage. Occasionally I would come out and ask to smell someone's food. They would often ask how I could stand that. Some people on the program said that smelling their favorite foods drove them crazy. Somehow, the smell satisfied me temporarily, and I got a vicarious thrill out of seeing people enjoy their food.

And yet people couldn't win with me. I was still squirrelly psychologically. If people complimented me, I felt good. If they were too effusive, I wondered what they must have thought of me when I was fat. If they said nothing, I felt neglected.

If someone in the family cavalierly ate something delicious in front of me, I might bark at them. "How can you be that insensitive when you know I'm not eating?"

But if they said, "Will it bother you if I have a sandwich?" I would snap, "Of course not! Why would it bother me? You think I can't handle it?" I was one wild and crazy guy. I knew I was irrational and borderline nuts, and I was grateful the family cut me some slack.

The highest compliment anyone could pay me was to simply act amazed at my discipline and willpower. Secretly, of course, I was still telling myself that the hard part was yet to come and that having virtually no decisions to make about food made the modified fast almost too easy.

Staying on it and succeeding was an accomplishment, of course. But I was justly worried about the future, afraid of real food, and wondering how I would do on the life-long hard part. Fortunately for me, I discovered some window-opening secrets about working out and about keeping track of what I ate.

Now hear me. If you haven't taken anything away from this book so far, I want you to know that I can empathize with you if both those areas sound so distasteful that they could be deal breakers. I don't know how many times I heard other people in the program say, "I'm just not the type to keep track of everything. It wouldn't be worth it. I'm not that analytical, and that's no way to live." They eventually crashed and burned. That's no way to live either.

But even more daunting, especially to a person who has battled weight a whole lifetime, is the idea of working out regularly. This was the place where I usually shut other diet books. Like anyone else, I wanted to be thin and healthy and active and feeling great. But exercise appeared too high a price.

I know well that that's where you may be on this subject right now. The idea of parking as far from an entrance as you can, rather than as close, or of taking stairs instead of an elevator, or actually *wanting* to walk or bicycle somewhere instead of riding in a car is as incomprehensible as if I began writing in some language from outer space.

Trust me, I was there. Yes, I speak now like a true convert, but I haven't forgotten. All I can do at this point is to plead with you to hear me out. You knew long-term results weren't going to be easy. But they *can* be fun (stay with me), and you *can* do it. So don't write anything off until you've heard it.

18

Doing It for Yourself

I make no guarantees that the same motivation will work for you, but something finally pushed me over the hump in this area of exercise. And I was not an easy sell.

Despite the fact that I grew up an athlete, nothing appealed to me less than an exercise regimen. That reminded me of gym class, calisthenics, workout programs on TV. Borrriiing!

For people who have never been athletic—no sports or games of any kind—exercising must look even worse. They must imagine themselves looking out of shape, uncoordinated, embarrassed. You think of aerobics classes where half the people are hard-bodied young men and women off the covers of magazines and the other half are middle-aged men and women out of their element, sweating more from embarrassment and humiliation than from activity.

So what finally motivated me? Memories and statistics.

My memories were not pleasant ones, and, because I still had the weight when I was considering all this, they weren't just memories of the distant past. These were memories I was still living and making. What did I remember?

- Hobbling when I first got up in the morning
- Short-term memory loss

- ✔ Lack of concentration
- ✔ An occasional attack of gout
- ✔ Being immobile
- ✔ Shortness of breath after a short flight of stairs
- ✔ Always having to watch rather than participate in anything that looked fun
- ✔ Feeling the need to explain my eating habits
- ✔ People saying "helpful" things
- ✔ Having to walk farther than expected and then suffering from excruciating bone spurs for six months, wondering if I would forever be an invalid
- ✔ Looking as if I was being born when simply extracting myself from behind the wheel of my car
- ✔ Looking for chairs without arm rests so that I could sit in, rather than appear to be wearing, the chair
- ✔ Having to buy my clothes at specialty shops with names like Eddie's Fashions for Behemoth Dudes

Those memories are only wryly humorous now. They're not funny when you're living them. The statistics weren't funny either.

When I finally got serious about taking off the weight and keeping it off, I knew there would be no magic, no secrets, and few surprises. I would have to finally cave in and sacrifice somewhere. There would be no miracle, fat-burning pill you take in the morning that allows you to sit all day eating candy and nuts and still see those pounds melt away.

No, the statistics I heard were ominous. Besides the fact that a mere 4 percent of the people who lose as much as I had to lose keep it off for more than a year, get this: 100 percent (you read that right) of the 4 out of 100 who *are* successful remain actively engaged in a regular exercise program. And they continue to keep food diaries, most of them for the rest of their lives.

Now, I know food diaries can seem more daunting than exercising, and if I hadn't found an easy and fun way to do it, that may have been my downfall. I'll get to that later, but let me try to win you over on exercise or you might as well close this book now.

Don't do that, tempting as it is. We all look for that one reason that disqualifies us. Stay with me. You've come too far. You were just getting psyched, so don't cash it in now. I'll make this as brief, as pedestrian, as persuasive, and as easy as possible. You don't have to be a jock to make it work. I like simple, handy tricks as much as anyone, and there are many possibilities for doing what you have to do to make exercise effective for you.

Here's the deal: All the experts say that for good cardio-vascular health—in other words, a sound heart—we need to get our pulse into what's called the *target heart zone* (THZ) for at least twenty minutes a day, three days a week. That's minimum. Even if you're not a math whiz, and I'm not, THZ is easy to figure.

Regardless of your weight, everyone starts with the arbitrary figure of 220. Subtract your age. For me, at this writing, that's 43, so the remainder is 177. That, theoretically, is my maximum heart rate. In other words, if I were on a treadmill going as hard and as long as I could, my heart rate might reach the high 170s. That is very strenuous and can be dangerous if maintained for long. The more out of shape I am, the quicker my heart would escalate to that range to keep up with my exertion.

HOW TO FIND YOUR TARGET HEART ZONE (THZ)

$220 - age$ = **Maximum heart rate (MHR)**

MHR $\times$ **.60** = **THZ low point**

MHR $\times$ **.70** = **THZ midpoint**

MHR $\times$ **.80** = **THZ high point**

When I took my initial treadmill test (a week or so into the all-liquid modified fast), it took just a few minutes to reach that heart rate. I weighed well over 300 pounds and had not worked out systematically for years. It took so long for my heart rate to return to normal that they were able to run all kinds of tests on me at an elevated pulse.

Nowadays, after eighteen months of regular aerobic exercise, I assume that it would take a long time and a lot of strenuous treadmill work to get my heart rate to maximum and that I would recover so quickly that tests would be difficult.

But that maximum heart rate you just figured (or should have) is only a reference point. If you're not being medically tested and carefully monitored, you don't want your pulse to ever be that high—with the possible exception of your having to react in an emergency and run for your life or do something superhuman.

Now take your maximum heart rate and multiply it by 60 percent, 70 percent, and 80 percent. For me, those figures come out to approximately 106, 124, and 142. My target heart zone is between 106 and 142 beats per minute, and 124 is the exact midpoint.

Most experts agree that there needs to be a warm up and a cool down period, so the time for those activities must be added to the twenty minutes of harder work while the pulse is in the THZ. Already you can see that you're looking at at least thirty minutes a day, three days a week. Four days is even better.

Ironically, the longer you engage in exercise that gets your pulse into the THZ, the better shape you get into and the harder you have to work to keep it there. That sounds daunting right now, but there's such a sense of accomplishment and well-being at that point that it will be worth it when you get there. Meanwhile, a few quick hints:

It's likely you know all this and have heard it or read it many times before. At the risk of being didactic, let me lay it out again from the perspective of one who had to battle all the psychological reasons to avoid the work. I don't come at this from the perspective of a lean young thing who's telling you that you will become sexy and alluring. I'm a middle-aged man who carried way too much weight for way too long and am finally succeeding at maintaining a loss. Exercise is a major, major key that can help you succeed too.

Like all the other diet and exercise advocates, I encourage you to get your doctor's approval for an exercise program. Unless you have some chronic ailment or disease, there is hardly a doctor anywhere who will discourage exercise in some format. If you are otherwise relatively healthy, except for your weight, you should be able to begin, albeit slowly.

That was one of the toughest things for me. Having been an athlete, I wanted to jump in and excel at some activity for half an hour or more and see immediate results. I'm glad I listened to counsel to start slowly and to give the program a month before deciding whether I saw any differences.

Here's my recommendation, depending on your preferences: If you're the type who needs a partner or even a group setting, find a Y or a local school or park district program and join an exercise club or aerobics class. If you are a private person and want to do this in the seclusion of your own home, you might invest in an aerobic video or two. Be sure to see samples before you buy. Some may have music that does nothing for you or have exercises inappropriate for where you're starting.

If you are indeed just starting out at this, be sure to begin with low-impact aerobics or an exercise bike, rather than high-impact aerobic dancing or a stepper or stair machine. You will quickly become sore and discouraged and may even injure yourself.

I started with an exercise bike, and, though it is not crucial, I recommend getting as many monitoring devices as you can afford. You should be able to gauge and record your time, distance, heart rate, calories burned, and whatever else interests you. That's the only way to know you're progressing.

The first few days on an exercise bike will make you wonder why you ever took my advice. The first few revolutions, at an easy setting, will seem a cinch and may even be fun. "Not bad," you'll tell yourself, and then you may overdo it. A family member may mosey past, and you'll show off how fast you can go. You'll regret that and pay for it the next day when you can hardly walk.

Trust me, all you're looking for the first few times on the bike are coordination and a slightly elevated heart rate. That should come quickly. If you can afford it, get a pulse monitor. Some of these attach to your earlobe or even to your chest or wrist. They can cost between $50 and $100, and they are not necessary if you know how to accurately check your own pulse. The drawback to taking your own pulse is that generally you have to stop walking or riding or whatever you're doing to get an accurate reading, and thus the reading is slightly skewed.

You can take your pulse by pressing two fingers lightly on your wrist, just below your hand on almost a direct line down from your thumb. It takes some experimenting to find the right spot to feel your pulse, and be careful not to press too hard because you can interrupt the flow of blood and affect the reading.

I almost always take my pulse—if manually—by placing thumb and finger at the pressure points in my neck, just below my jaw on either side. The drawback here is that the thumb also has a pulse, but that has never seemed to throw me off. If you take your pulse at your neck it becomes even more important not to press too hard. You can actually cause yourself to pass out if you stop the flow of blood there.

Determining whether you're in your target heart zone is fairly simple. Merely count your heartbeats for 10 seconds and multiply by 6, or for 15 seconds and multiply by 4. If your pulse for 10 seconds is 15, that multiplied by 6 is 90. If your resting pulse rate is in the 70 range, you know your pulse is elevated and getting you warmed up.

After a few minutes of exercise, especially involving your largest muscles—those in your legs—your pulse should gradually increase. If you're my age, you want to see your heart rate get into the lower end of the THZ (106 +) and gradually start climbing toward 140 or so. When my 10-second pulse rate is at about 12, I'm right in the middle of my THZ.

As I mentioned, the newer you are to exercise, the quicker your pulse will rise. You may find, especially if you start too quickly, that your heart will zoom past your THZ in the first couple of minutes. That is a clue that you have begun much too quickly. Don't stop, unless you feel pain or discomfort, but slow down and let your pulse settle into your THZ.

To give you a hint of how things change once you get into shape, consider that it takes me between eight and twelve minutes of fairly vigorous riding on a stationary bike now to get into the lower range of my THZ. By the twenty-minute mark I am in the upper region and can maintain that for several more minutes. My recovery time—that is, seeing my pulse return to under a hundred and start dropping to my normal resting rate (which is now about 60)—can be as little as two to three minutes. When I began, my pulse would stay in the nineties for up to half an hour after a workout.

If you invest in an apparatus such as a stationary cycle, you might want to ride as little as five to seven minutes the first day, skip the next, ride another five to seven, skip, then ride another five to seven. You'll feel a little achiness the day after, but you will be amazed at how quickly you build endurance.

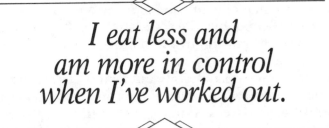

I eat less and am more in control when I've worked out.

That first day you may be huffing and puffing and seeing your pulse skyrocket, and you'll think I'm crazy for suggesting that someday you'll be pedaling away for thirty to sixty minutes at a time. Don't give up too soon. You'll get impatient for results, but they will come. Those results will seem insignificant at first. They will probably entail your realizing that you can ride fifteen minutes, or twenty, with less discomfort. Your heart will enjoy the workout. It'll take you longer to get your pulse up, which means you're getting into shape.

You may actually miss the workout on your off days (that is a *real* step). You'll find you're walking and moving more easily at other times of the day. The exercise may release endorphins in your brain that give you a sense of well-being and confidence. If the bike bores you, move into aerobics, walking, a stepper, cycling outside, racquetball, tennis, basketball, or—if you're young and healthy and light enough—even jogging. That's not for me, but it sure is a great aerobic workout. I love variety and I love to compete, but I have to make sure that my activity keeps me in my target heart zone *constantly* during the workout.

Now, I can't hide the fact that here is a bit of bad news, depending on how you look at it. A half hour or so of aerobic work every other day, getting your pulse into the target heart zone for at least twenty of those minutes, will have little effect on your weight or the percentage of fat in your body. You'll burn off a few calories, yes, and that may even curb your appetite. (Many believe that exercise makes you hungrier, but try it for yourself. I eat less and am more in control when I've worked out—generally before breakfast because it seems to jump start my metabolism and helps my body process my food more efficiently.) Such a workout is wonderful for your heart and should be the minimum you do to help you maintain your loss.

But, if you want to literally burn fat and really excise calories, you want to work up to a vigorous, more lengthy exercise several days a week. I'm not saying mine is the only way to do it, but let me give you an idea of my program.

I am still a high-volume eater. I have cut my fat percentages to the low twenties per day (from probably around the 50 percent range in the past) and my calories dramatically, but I am not on a restricted, low-calorie diet. I can eat anything I want, as long as the fat content stays below 30 percent for the day and the total calories are no more than twelve times the pounds I weigh.

If I want to eat more, I must exercise, and, if I want to maintain or lose, I must burn fat. Experts such as Covert Bailey (*Fit or Fat*) and Richard Simmons (*Deal-A-Meal*) and others will tell you that real fat burning in exercise begins after the aerobic benefit has already taken place.

In other words, once you have warmed up and gotten your pulse into the THZ, the longer you stay at it, the more fat the body burns for fuel. In fact, they say that longer periods at the lower end of the THZ are better than shorter periods at the high end. I am at a point where it isn't unusual for me to spend an hour on the exercise bike or thirty to forty-five minutes on a stepper machine or an hour on the racquetball court (the least boring and the most fun) per day, six days a week. Richard

Simmons *never* takes a day off exercise. He says, "I eat every day, so I work out every day." I find I need that day off. I try to eat less that day but often find I eat more.

If you prefer swimming, that is great too. For some reason it is not the fat burner the other exercises are, but it is probably the best for a total body workout and for aerobic benefit. Whatever you decide upon, make sure it's something you can learn to enjoy and look forward to and that sustains your THZ. Lots of walking up and down stairs and doing housework or gardening is good, but it is no substitute. There are too many interruptions that make the heart rate plummet, and that costs you the benefit.

I am addicted to the endorphin rush produced by a good, long, sweaty workout. I feel great. I feel lighter, more motivated to stick to my diet. I am stronger, healthier, and even think more clearly.

To reduce the boredom factor, I always read or watch television while on the bike. I can't read on the stepper because I'm bobbing too much, but I have found I can watch the early morning news. Best of all, if my wife is doing an aerobic workout to an exercise video, I find that the music gets me into a rhythm, especially on the stepper, that makes my strenuous workout seem shorter and easier. That really burns the calories.

At my weight, I can burn a couple of thousand calories in an extended session on the stepper, and that allows me the occasional treat that would otherwise sabotage my program.

Best of all, if I learned nothing else from my weeks on the New Direction program, I somehow learned to quit being a perfectionist in this exercise area. If I miss a day or two—or even three, which rarely happens—I get right back to it. I know that even if I've lost the edge, if I've fallen a certain percentage out of shape and can't go as hard and fast and long as I did a few days before, anything I do is beneficial to me and my body and my diet right now. And so I do it.

At this writing I am out of commission temporarily with a knee injury. I still lift weights every other day—because building muscle burns fat and tones the body—and even though I have gone longer away from bike, stepper, or racquetball court than ever before in the last eighteen months, I will be back to my regular routine as soon as possible. No doubt my heart will race at first, and I may be able to go only twenty to thirty minutes the first few days. But there is not one iota of thought that I will thus give it up. I know the benefits, and I can't wait to get back and start reaping them.

If you're like I was, you can't imagine getting up at the crack of dawn (I need less sleep than ever now too), getting into workout clothes, and hitting a piece of equipment for thirty to sixty minutes before a shower and breakfast. Once you get started, however, you'll wonder how you ever got along without it.

You may not be able to get into the swing of it early in your weight loss program, depending on your weight and fitness. But start slowly, even with an occasional walk. Get used to moving more—and differently—as the weight comes off so that by the time you are adapting to your new body and lifestyle you are able to get serious about physical activity. Exercise is one of the two hallmarks of people who have successfully maintained significant weight losses.

The other characteristic is keeping a food diary, which can sound just as daunting as exercise. But there *is* a way to do it. Stay with me.

19

The Dreaded Diary

I confess that keeping track of everything I ate was a problem for me. In most of the diets I had been on over the years, this idea was espoused. Sometimes they even checked during the first few weeks to be sure we were keeping a diary. That was all well and good. Yes, it was always surprising to find out what I had been eating. Rarely can you keep up without recording every amount.

I don't know why I didn't like that part of it, but my guess is that you wouldn't either. Too much writing. Too much work. It's a nuisance. It's sometimes depressing. It doesn't necessarily keep you from overeating, and then you're tempted to be less than honest in your own food diary. Lying to ourselves has always been part of our problem, so getting cute with a diary is another step on the road to failure.

When I finally found the system that has made a food diary work for me, I made an absolute commitment to be honest with it. I rationalize nothing. As you will see later, I still cheat. I still eat things I shouldn't. I still have my days, my failures, my frustrations. But I will not hide them from my record-keeping program. If I binge, I record it. I may self-defeatingly talk myself into eating food that destroys my whole day and somehow temporarily convince myself I won't regret it (which I always do), but I will live with it in my food diary. My occasional super-high calorie day, that high fat thing I couldn't resist, all get recorded and added to my totals and averages.

When I was keeping track of what I consumed while on the modified fast, it was interesting and exciting because I was doing so well. I had only what I was allowed, so I dutifully recorded my four protein drinks and their 880 calories, my hundreds of ounces (yes) of water and diet, caffeine-free drinks per day, and my fewer than a hundred calories of sugar-free diet Jell-O.

It was exciting, and I was proud to keep track of that little amount. But as I looked forward to my first real food, I dreaded keeping track of lettuce leaves, ounces of chicken, pieces of fruit, and all that. I knew it was important, and I committed myself to doing it. But I couldn't imagine that for the rest of my life. I tried to put it into the category of exercise, which I did at first medicinally, then grew to enjoy and see as a major element in my success. But keeping track of *everything*? It would keep me honest, sure, but what a drag.

Well, that first meal came and went. I opted for three ounces of shrimp—which looked like a huge feast—on a bed of lettuce with some fat-free dressing. The whole family waited with bated breath to see if I could swallow. I enjoyed it immensely but with some trepidation, fearing it would trigger an appetite I couldn't control. I did look forward to my next real food, which was a day away (I was still on the beverage, substituting a small meal for one drink each week for the next four weeks), and I was encouraged that I continued to lose.

Right about that time I got a piece of direct mail from a computer software company, Parsons Technology. It contained a brochure for a program called the Diet Analyst. A satisfied customer said he had used the program to keep track of his eating and even his meal planning and had lost two pounds a week for a year on his own.

I didn't need to lose, but I needed to maintain, and this looked like the solution. It was fairly inexpensive, so I ordered it. At the risk of sounding like a commercial, I have to tell you—it has become a major element in my success. The program, with frequent updates, very simply includes most of the foods you'll find anywhere, many of them by brand name, including fast foods. And if a food does not appear on its list, you can add it if it has an ingredients label. You simply tap in the information and it's there forever.

You plug in your name, age, sex, height, weight, what you would like to weigh, whether you want to maintain or lose one or two pounds a week, and whether your activity level is light, moderate, or heavy. I chose light, despite my workouts, because exercise is figured separately. If you both exercise and work construction or are a professional athlete, you would select the heavy activity level. All that figures into the program's suggested calorie counts and nutritional percentages for you.

Everything is adjustable too. For instance, when I bounced the figures off the New Direction staff, they suggested that I could increase my sodium and cholesterol intake limits based on my own medical profile.

Then, based on all the factors I plugged in, the Diet Analyst program listed goals and limits for me. It told me how many calories I should have per day and what percentage of those should come from protein, carbohydrate, and fat. Every day I bring my file up on the computer screen and tap in what I have eaten, merely highlighting the foods and entering them by a few keystrokes from simple lists. The program automatically computes the calories, the protein, carbohydrate, fat (saturated, monounsaturated, and polyunsaturated), cholesterol, fiber, caffeine, and sixteen other vitamins and nutrients.

It prints out a listing of the percentages of daily requirements, the actual intake measured in grams, and whether the levels were high, low, or OK. An ancillary program includes every food ingredient available, so even your own recipes can be added to the menus. Today, no matter what I eat, I can either find it in Diet Analyst or add it.

If this sounds complex, believe me it's not. I know only enough about computers to hit the right keys. I can't program, and I don't have a clue as to why the keys do what they do. But if you can add two and two and make yes or no decisions, you can make use of the Diet Analyst almost in your sleep.

Even if you've never worked on a computer, if you own one or someone in your house uses one, you can install Diet Analyst (or another comparable diet program) on it and have a simple, fun tool that makes keeping food diaries easy. I can print out my intake daily, weekly, or even up to two months at a time. It gives totals, percentages, and averages. Whether I'm gaining, losing, or maintaining, I can quickly see why from this program.

But there is a feature on it that is even better than its fun and ease of use. I work at my computer all day every day, so it's easy for me to just click over to the Diet Analyst after every meal or snack, but the best feature is that it allows me to plan ahead.

For instance, this morning I had a breakfast that included Ultra Slim Fast Plus (because I like the flavor, the bulk, and the fact that because of my size and weight I am allowed a double dose of it). To that I added two ounces of All Bran (one ounce of extra fiber and one ounce of original), three cups of skim milk, and ice cubes, and I blended it all into a large shake.

That gave me a breakfast containing more than 100 percent of all the vitamins and nutrients I'll need for the whole day and much more fiber than I require. I don't happen to like All Bran as a bowl of cereal with milk and artificial sweetener, but I do enjoy it as part of my breakfast shake.

Now, if I for some reason don't eat my fruits and vegetables as I should, I'll still have all the ingredients I need in my body for health. If I stray from my diet and eat something higher in fat, the low fat content of that breakfast will average it out. But back to the program and this great feature.

I plugged in the breakfast, which is easy because the program gives me the capability of combining common ingredients. Since I often have such a breakfast, I combined the two servings of Ultra Slim Fast Plus with the three cups of skim milk and the two ounces of All Bran and named it USFP AB Mix. Now I can enter all those ingredients with one key stroke.

Another key brings up a screen that tells me that if twenty-five minutes of lifting (which is nonaerobic, by the way) is the only exercise I do today, my breakfast has given me 27 percent of my daily calories. I've had just 4 percent of my cholesterol limit for the day, 130 percent of my fiber, 0 percent caffeine, and well over 100 percent of vitamins A, C, D, E, B_6, and B_1, as well as riboflavin, niacin, folate, calcium, magnesium, potassium, iron, and zinc. (I confess I don't know what more than half of those are, why they're important, or what they mean. But I figure that if they are all kept at their proper daily levels, I don't have to worry about them.)

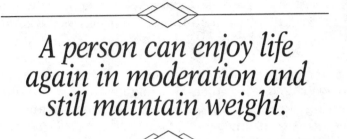

A person can enjoy life again in moderation and still maintain weight.

The Diet Analyst also shows that I'm still within my sodium range and that 20 percent of my calories have come from protein, 75 percent from carbohydrates, and 5 percent from fat (well under my 30 percent guideline and my norm of about 21 percent).

So what's so great about being able to plan ahead, which I do every day? Let's say I really have a taste for pizza today. Yes, pizza. People are always shocked to see me enjoying pizza. "I didn't know you could have that," they say, as if it's their business. (We'll get into that later.) But, yes, compulsive overeaters with weight problems can work pizza into their daily program if they have a handle on their totals.

Just for fun, let's say I have a Pizza Hut personal pan pizza for lunch and a thirty-two-ounce Diet Pepsi to help fill me up. Sure, I should be having a salad with fat-free dressing, but I'm trying to show here that a person can enjoy life again in moderation and still maintain weight.

The Diet Analyst tells me that I am now at 1,284 calories for the day, or 55 percent of my total allowance. That's great, because it allows for a low-fat frozen yogurt dessert, like a couple of cones from McDonald's. Sounds decadent and ridiculous, but this planning feature in Diet Analyst lets me know if it's permissible and what it will do to my totals.

My fat percentage has jumped to 16 percent because of the pizza, but that's still well within my limits. The large Diet Pepsi has added 38 percent of my daily allowance of caffeine, something I wouldn't do after 6:00 P.M. because I'm not a coffee drinker and have no tolerance for caffeine. It is a natural diuretic, and it is also a stimulant that will keep me awake. I keep plenty of caffeine-free diet pop on hand for dinner and after.

Some people would have to watch the sodium levels of the food I've had so far, and smaller men and most women would be getting close to their daily limits of calories and fats. But you could also cut my totals in half and see that you're still far from deprived on this program.

The low-fat yogurt cones at McDonald's are lifesavers for me. After having been able to stay off sugar for months at a time when I was on a high-calorie and high-fat diet in the past, for some reason I suffered from an insatiable sweet tooth when I got off the modified fast. The people at New Direction strongly recommended working sweets into my daily plan rather than eliminating them altogether. Because I'm diabetic I had to keep an eye on my blood sugar levels, but, because I was keeping the weight off and exercising, I found I could handle the extra sugar. It also kept me from bingeing on half a cake or a bag of cookies after weeks of deprivation.

I can't, of course, have what I really want: real ice cream —the rich, thick, creamy, fat-laden stuff—unless I want half a cup a day. Forget that! Those cones at McDonald's are 100 calories each and only 6.3 percent fat! Yes, they are empty, sugar-filled calories, and I would do better to have a piece of fruit or a salad. But I'm talking reality here. You and I are scrambling to maintain weight loss and keep from bingeing and messing up the whole deal. If having a personal pan pizza from Pizza Hut and yogurt cones from McDonald's is possible by having the kind of breakfast I outlined, I'm glad to be able to do it.

I know that the natural fibers in fruits are better than something added to cereal. And I know that the vitamins and nutrients in natural foods are better than those infused into diet shakes. But at times of desperation we look for what will tide us over and work until we can get a handle on what has sabotaged us in the past. I work well in a regimented program where I know what I'm getting out of everything I'm eating.

As I look at my Diet Analyst after the breakfast and lunch and dessert I enjoyed, I see that the cones have added 200 calories and dropped my fat percentage for the day to 15. I still have 36 percent of my daily calorie allowance left for dinner and a snack. It may not be the healthiest, but, if I wanted a treat like popcorn, I could probably fit it into the total.

Generally, I try to avoid more fats when I've had pizza or a McLean burger at McDonald's. Though I might be able to get away with it, I find that I maintain or lose more easily if I enjoy a higher fat item only once a day. So there won't be pizza *plus* a McLean. There won't be chicken *and* beef, pizza *and* popcorn. (Another fast-food hint: the BK Broiler chicken sandwich at Burger King is tasty and well within calorie and fat percentage limits if you order it without the sauce. I enjoy it that way, but you can add fat-free dressing or whatever fits your plan. Fast-food places don't have to be off-limits for everything but salads. When you're tired of feeling as if you're the only person in the family on a diet, try some of these more normal selections, which you have analyzed in advance.)

Certain candies are very low in fat, things such as Twizzlers or Skittles or Circus Peanuts. Stay away from the chocolate candy bars. You might be able to get away with one (for instance a Snickers Bar) as a substitute for a meal, but then you'll really have to watch your fats and total calories in everything else.

Now, make no mistake: I realize that it would be foolhardy to recommend pizza and frozen yogurt and popcorn and candy as general staples of a maintenance diet. But can you see that occasionally you may have a day like that, not feeling deprived or hungry, and still stay within your calorie and fat percentage limits?

I love the planning feature on Diet Analyst because it allows me to see what's coming. I hardly ever eat what I have planned, but I usually eat the equivalent. I may have planned a nice supper of a couple of those healthy frozen dinners that contain 250-300 calories each. But as dinnertime approaches I may get a craving for something sweet or cold. I can have that if I eliminate one or both of those dinners. It may not be quite as healthy in the long run, but by planning I have stayed within my totals. And I've certainly eaten healthier than I did when I was gorging on cheeseburgers and not working out at all.

If you have the willpower and stamina to eat the right things all the time, you may not need these gimmicks or this book. But if you're like me and you eventually start feeling sorry for yourself, you could be headed for bingeing problems and long-term failures.

You probably know by now how to read labels and determine fat percentages. But in case you don't and because, either way, this gives me the chance to editorialize on the sleazy tactics of some food processors, let me summarize it for you.

For some reason, probably because the public has become so fat conscious, food producers list calories in hard numbers and fats in grams. So, if you see a food that says one serving is just 100 calories and only 6 grams of fat, you might think, *Hey, great!*

But here's the problem. Every gram of fat represents 9 calories. Sounds complicated, but it isn't. Just remember that every time you see fat grams listed they have to be multiplied by 9. If you can't multiply by 9 easily, round it up to 10. That's close enough, and all you have to do is add a zero to the number. Then you divide the fat calories by the total and you get the percentage of fat. Also remember that the "one serving" on the label is sometimes ridiculously small. Depending on how much you actually plan to eat, you may have to increase the calorie count even more.

If you're trying to keep your fat percentage under 30 a day, that means that your calories from fat have to *average out* below 30 percent. Thus, if you decide to eat something well *above* 30 percent, you have to eat something else equal in calories that is well *below* 30 percent. That product I mentioned that was 100 calories per serving and just 6 grams of fat is, *ta da*, 54 percent fat! If you're eating only Slim Fast shakes or sawdust the rest of the day, you might be able to work it in.

If, for instance, you wanted to have a Snickers Bar, you would punch it up on your computer and find this: In a mere 2.1 ounces you have 270 calories and 12.7 grams of fat. Multiply those grams by 9, and you get 114 calories from fat, or 42 percent. If you can work it in, work it in. But consider: Does

162

such a candy bar trigger cravings and eating patterns that have done you in in the past? Is it worth it? Can you discipline yourself to have just one? You might rather have three cones at McDonald's for 30 more calories than the candy, a lot more bulk, and a fraction of the fat.

If you absolutely *have* to have a chocolate candy bar, talk yourself into a Milky Way. It has only 9.8 grams of fat, or 88.2 calories, about 33 percent of the 270 total calories. Better yet, enjoy the Skittles or the Twizzlers. All this from one easy computer program.

Keeping track and planning ahead have become indispensable and fun for me. I plan when I'm traveling and often find I do better on the road than at home. I regiment myself. Recently I was gone for three days and was unable to work out because of my knee injury. With the program I limited my calories and fat percentages, taking into consideration my eliminated exercise.

I was feeling particularly deprived because my calorie intake had been cut by at least 500 a day. So I enjoyed my pizza and my McLeans and my yogurt cones. I've eaten more healthfully, but during my temporary physical setback this carried me. After having worked out strenuously six days a week for more than a year, suddenly I was immobile. Yet, because I worked at it and planned ahead, I actually lost more than two pounds during that week, and because I was enjoying foods that have become treats I didn't feel deprived.

Traveling can be difficult because there is often down time and private time when no one would know what you were eating. I recall going to a convention after I had first lost my weight, fearing that I would enjoy the public accolades and then self-destruct by being a problem eater alone via room service.

Rather, I set a goal not just to keep from gaining, not just to maintain, but actually to lose weight. I told my comrades in my sustaining class and determined to use room service to my advantage. One of the women said, "We'll be pulling for you." What an encouragement that was! And how often I thought of it when I was tempted to eat unwisely that week.

I took my sweats and my pulse monitor and exercised in the hotel workout room every morning. (That's something else that will surprise you when you get in shape. You won't be embarrassed to work out in public. It can actually make you justifiably proud that you can handle a piece of equipment and look like you know what you're doing, working up a sweat and keeping track of your progress. People who work out recognize strangers who do the same. You can tell by the muscle tone and the healthy skin color.)

I used room service wisely. I took my notebook computer and looked up the foods in the menu. Then I planned ahead to eat healthy, tasty stuff, including a few treats. I lost a pound that week and took a huge step in self-confidence.

20

The Self Factor

Something you may have sensed by now is that maintaining a significant weight loss is serious business. It requires time. It also requires something that we Christians feel guilty about: a preoccupation with ourselves. It's not that we don't naturally want to think about ourselves. We all want to and do, but we know we shouldn't. Or we think we shouldn't.

Certainly we shouldn't think of ourselves as more important or wonderful than we are. And clearly we should not think of ourselves more highly than we do of others. That's the biblical ideal. On the other hand, God knows our frame and remembers that we are dust (Psalm 103:14). He knows we love ourselves in spite of our self-image problems. We may disgust ourselves, but we still serve ourselves. That's why Scripture tells us over and over that we are to love our neighbors as we love ourselves. Lest you think that admonition is found only once, check out these references in their contexts: Leviticus 19:18; Matthew 19:19; 22:39; Mark 12:31; 12:33; Romans 13:9; and James 2:8.

Such a command may sound strange to those of us with weight problems. At our core, we have self-doubt. We hide. We cover. We retreat. We erect barriers. We don't like ourselves too much.

But there is a dichotomy here, which I will get to when I discuss what I have discovered about the whys of self-destructive behavior when we know better. The dichotomy is that for all our alleged self-loathing, there is also a prodigious preoccupation with our wants and needs.

On the modified fast, I found that all I could think about was food. I had no physical hunger after a while, but the mouth hunger (the taste for things) and the mental hunger (the missing of the fun and fellowship of eating with others, of something to look forward to) were overwhelming. I drove my friends and family crazy talking about food, diets, programs, fasts, recipes, and plans to eat when I finally could.

Even when I got back on food, I obsessed about it. To be able to plan once again for meals became huge in my mind. Exercising, keeping food diaries, thinking about all the above, and plotting against my nature to maintain my loss made me so self-possessed that even I got tired of me.

I still see some of that. Perhaps getting it on paper will be cathartic and I can give it a rest, but of course there is the possibility that this will merely create more interest and give me more of a platform to yak about it.

In spite of all that, let me encourage you to invest in yourself. Spend the money it takes to immerse yourself in a reducing plan that is healthy and that works. Make sure it's one that emphasizes adapting and maintenance and doesn't merely give lip service to the dreaded "change of lifestyle" or the "change of eating habits." Sometimes I think if I hear that one more time from some well-meaning civilian I'm going to explode.

I know full well that I have indeed changed my lifestyle (working out, keeping track of what I eat) and my eating habits (consuming slightly less volume and dramatically fewer calories), but the prospect of that did not motivate me to change in the least. When someone heard about my reducing plan and said, "Now what you need is a complete change of lifestyle," I nodded politely.

But that sounded to me just like it does to you. What do they think our lifestyle consists of? Do they think we eat constantly? That we live to eat rather than eat to live? (Bet you've heard that more than once!) Grief, I hated those references to "complete" changes, as if I should now start eating with silverware rather than with my hands and, perish the thought, chewing before swallowing. Not too overly sensitive, was I?

You will find, however, that real progress is made only through carving out time for yourself. No one else is going to do this for you. You will feel selfish, and you may even be accused of the same. If you were doing this only to make yourself more attractive or assertive or successful, maybe you *should* feel guilty. But I am not one of those who says, "You've spent enough time living for everyone else; it's time to do something for you." That is too modern, too narcissistic.

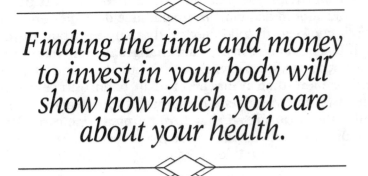

Finding the time and money to invest in your body will show how much you care about your health.

But you are going to find that to do anything right and well and lasting you will need to give yourself to it. That same drive that has made you good at whatever it is you're good at—whether that's being a spouse, a parent, a professional, a creator, a student—is required to make you successful at maintaining your weight.

We find time to do what we really want to do. People who are late to church are never late to a movie. People who are late for appointments always seem to get to the ball game on time.

We find the money to do what we really want to do. People who can't afford to be generous find the funds for that vacation. People who can't give systematically to God's work find the money for that new car.

Finding the time and money to invest in your body will show how much you care about your health. I have found that healthy eating is a little more expensive and that keeping track of what I eat and working out costs me more than an extra hour each day. If my health and my future were not worth that to me, I would decide that I couldn't afford the time or the money. It's a matter of priorities. Some things have to go, and what you choose to sacrifice will reveal how important your health really is to you.

Seriously, if you decide it's not worth the effort, that's your call. I'm not going to be the one to judge and say your priorities are distorted. But I would urge you not to complain about your weight or your health and to quit talking about what you should do about it, if you have decided—and proven by your choices—that it is not really that important to you.

If you've read this far, such changes *are* important to you. As one who has been trying to live out that kind of commitment for more than two years, I want to encourage you to set aside the time you need to maintain your weight loss. You should not be surprised that it requires a time commitment. I've found the time it takes more than worth it.

A Special Two-Chapter
Section for Civilians

21

What to Say to a Fat Person

There is nothing wrong with your book. This chapter has been left intentionally blank. Get it?

22

What Not to Say to a Fat Person

"Your face is your redeeming feature."
Thanks. Your mouth is not yours.
"Wouldn't you feel better if you did something about your weight?"
Better about what? About what my friends say to me and about me?
"Are you doing anything about your weight?"
Just eating, thanks.
"When are you going to do something about your weight?"
When you stop asking.
"Should I be eating this in front of you?"
No. Get thee behind me.
"Should you be eating that?"
Maybe not, Mother. What do you think I should eat?
"Have you tried eating just one helping of everything and having fruit for dessert?"
You mean food has something to do with this? In a lifetime of obesity, I never thought of that.
"I told my kids that if they didn't behave I'd have you sit on them."
Apparently you love them as much as you do me.
"How much do you weigh?"
How old are you?

"Are you really still hungry?"
I try to stay ahead of hunger. I haven't been hungry for years.
"Have you tried the [your choice here] diet?"
I can't imagine having missed it.

I know that the italicized responses are mean spirited. I have never said anything like that out loud, but you can bet I've thought them frequently because I've heard such comments and questions more times than I care to count.

We who battle with our weight and our eating habits know, somewhere way down deep, that you mean well. We really do. The problem is that we are so supersensitive that we interpret every helpful remark as a sign of conditional acceptance. If you honestly think we don't know why we're fat or how to lose or how to maintain, you are hurling the most cutting insult. But even all those kind remarks you make with the purest of motives wound us.

Of course, many comments *are* meant to be cruel. But most, I'm sure, are not. You really want to help, and you don't know what to say. Say nothing. Please. We know we're fat. We know we appear undisciplined. We know we seem stupid for still eating when we are unhappy with ourselves. We know what will make us fat and what will make us thin. Knowing isn't the point.

Your help doesn't help. It makes us feel worse. It implies that we would be more acceptable to you if we would change. We would embarrass you less or gain your respect. Even your compliments when we do succeed—and, of course, we love those—must be tempered with the knowledge that we are fragile people, despite our bulk. Notice our achievement, yes, but exult too much about your new admiration and respect and we will irrationally (we hope) assume that when we were overweight, you neither admired nor respected us—and certainly you didn't love us unconditionally.

I know we're asking too much. We're asking that you exhibit the unconditional love of God. That's not fair of us, and though it may seem we are wallowing in self-pity when this is a state we have brought on ourselves, consider: If you really, really want to help, give us the benefit of the doubt.

We don't do this to ourselves on purpose, at least consciously. There is little you can tell us that we don't already know. Generally, whatever has contributed to making us this way also makes us incapable of sticking up for ourselves and telling you what we think of your comments.

Once a friend asked me sincerely how he could help. I trusted him enough to ask if he really wanted to know. He said yes. I said, "Ignore it. No comments, no looks, no faces, no shrugs, no catering, no enabling. Ignore it. It's my problem. I'm aware of it. I'm working on it, even when it appears I'm failing."

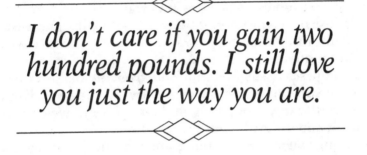

I don't care if you gain two hundred pounds. I still love you just the way you are.

Bless him, he appreciated my counsel and took it. After that exchange he knew he was not enabling me when he ignored it if I ate too much or ordered more. Had I been intimidated enough to eat less than I wanted in front of him, I would have resented it later and eaten even more than I wanted in private. It's sick and it's wrong, but there it is.

Even when someone you know raises the issue of his or her own weight problem, you must still be careful. Though he may be saying, "Really, I want your help," what he means is, "I want your unconditional love and support." In fact, if he insists that you tell him or remind him or "not allow" him something, you should refuse. Rather, you should say, "That is your business, and I know you can handle it yourself. I don't care if you gain two hundred pounds. I still love you just the way you are."

That often begins a dialogue fraught with danger for the sincere friend.

"But you want me thinner."

"I want you happy."

"But you want me healthy."

"Of course. I want you with me for as long as possible."

"So you think I'm eating myself to death."

"I think I want you healthy, like you said."

"You wish I weren't so fat."

"I love you just the way you are."

"But you know it would be better for me if I was thinner."

"I want you happy and healthy, but how you look and what you weigh has absolutely nothing to do with my love for you."

"But you don't respect me this way."

"I respect you enough to know that you can do whatever you set your mind to."

And it goes on. I've been on the wrong side of that conversation for years, and I'm telling you, from my perspective what the fat person wants is support and love. It may take you years to convince him you mean it, and one look or face or shrug or comment can undo all your protestations.

When you get past your patience and become parental and give the big speech ("You really must do something about your weight") you will open a chasm that may never close.

I know it sounds as if I'm saying that fat people want everyone to be enablers. I'm not. I'm saying that we know—believe me, we know. You love us, you care, you're sincere, you mean well, but your heartfelt counsel is driving us to private binges to cover the pain of knowing we are being judged by our failures.

Are we then blaming it on you? Only temporarily. Yes, we might binge anyway, for other reasons. Yes, we're feeling sorry for ourselves and finding yet another excuse to overeat. But, again, if you are sincere in wanting to help, let us deal with our problem our own way.

I have heard one account of a struggler asking her roommate to help in a tangible way, but that came with strict ground rules. She told her roommate, "If you see me with something I said I wasn't going to eat, you can ask me if I really want it. If I say yes, you can ask me if I'm sure, not in a scolding way, just informationally. If I still say yes, ignore me. If I really don't want it, one of those first two questions will remind me and I will decide against having it. But if I withstand that, don't give me a look. Just let me be. If I regret it later, so be it."

I know it's not easy and I know it's not fair. When your motives are pure and you're watching a friend or loved one self-destruct, it's almost impossible to hold your tongue. But you must, or you'll do more harm than good. It's not your fault. It's ours. But it is still true.

If you have nagged a spouse, a child (adult or otherwise), or anyone else about his or her weight, it's never too late to set the record straight. The one time they will accept input is when you have seen the light, whether you agree or understand or not.

I recommend saying or writing something like: "I have come to learn that my comments about your weight are not helpful. You may have tried to indicate that to me many times in many ways over the years, but I missed it. I want you to know that I meant well [resist the temptation to get in a little final sermonizing here], but I was wrong. No matter what you weigh or how you're doing on (or not doing on) any diet, I love you just the way you are and only want you happy and healthy. Of course, I know that you want the same. I will not raise the issue again, and I want you to forgive me for any insensitivity I have ever shown."

Two of the best comments I received from friends after my rather dramatic weight loss, one from a fellow struggler and one not, both communicated virtually the same thing. After congratulating me on the accomplishment, each said, "You know I love you either way."

Nothing could mean more or be more motivating than that. All that makes me want to do is to stay healthy. It doesn't give me license to fall off the wagon and suffer an extended lapse. It's that kind of support that brings me back from temporary failures, lapses, binges, and the like.

Yes, they still happen. And for the rest of the way I'd like to share what I've learned in my personal war thus far and the conclusions I've come to that may be of help to fellow strugglers.

23

What I've Learned

Despite my insistence that no one is more of an expert on weight loss and gain than the obese person, I have to admit that I have learned a lot through the New Direction program. I'll never forget telling behaviorist Sarah Bieber during that initial interview that I doubted I would learn anything new. In a sense, that has been true. In some form or other (articles, books, tapes, testimonials, personal experience) I have heard it all before. So have you.

- Avoid sugar.
- Don't eat between meals.
- Eat only when you're hungry.
- Don't allow yourself to become too hungry.
- Fill up on high fiber veggies.
- Drink lots of water and diet drinks.
- Eat balanced meals.
- Eat slowly, no second helpings.
- Avoid fats.
- Exercise.
- Think happy thoughts.

- ↙ Avoid dangerous situations.
- ↙ Envision yourself lean and trim.
- ↙ Get rid of the old fat wardrobe.
- ↙ Don't let dinner be the heaviest meal of the day.
- ↙ Don't eat before bedtime.

You can add a dozen more. We've all heard them. We all know them. No news, no revelations. They remind me of the title of that best-selling book *All I Really Need to Know I Learned in Kindergarten.*

Problem is, they don't work. Whoops, that almost slid past me. The problem isn't that *they* don't work. It's that *we* don't work. If we did all the above, we would be trim, flat, healthy, happy, robust, and successful.

Many, many people accomplish the above as a natural course. I know people to whom eating is incidental. Bruce Yamamoto, director of New Direction at Victory Hospital, is one. It's probably the only thing that should disqualify him from his job. He's compassionate, knowledgeable, thorough. He cares. He's learning to understand, but that has to be his biggest challenge. He once asked me, during a particularly difficult time in my maintenance program, whether I could simply use normal hunger as an eating signal.

I laughed, and he took it good naturedly when I told others in the program of the ridiculous thing he had said. To civilians —and I hate to lump Bruce, who has been so instrumental to my success, with civilians—eating when you're hungry and stopping when you're satisfied seems the most natural thing in the world (that's why they are civilians). I know people who can stop midway through a Whopper sandwich and leave the rest because they're no longer hungry.

Hungry? What's hunger got to do with it?!

Late in my fast, with just a couple of weeks to go, I was sailing along. I had not cheated and I would not. I was at a point where I could even sit at parties with people and enjoy (believe it or not) watching them munch on some of my favorite foods. I was at a family retreat and had had my beverage. People around me were eating pizza. One woman had two slices on her plate. I didn't think much of it until I noticed that she ate one and ignored the other.

Truthfully, it was not a temptation for me. It would be today, now that I am back on food. I would likely find some way to justify working it into my total program. But what struck me back then, when I was off solid foods, was that I simply could not comprehend leaving good food.

Had I been raised in poverty or been hungry as a child or deprived, I could understand that. How I envied this woman! But more than that, I was dumbfounded. I tried and tried to get my mind around that. I knew beyond doubt that even if I was stuffed to the point of discomfort, I would not have left a piece of pizza.

Can you identify with that? Do you wish I had some magic answer that explains it? So do I, because the conclusions I have come to are dark and ugly. But, before I get to those, I need to tell you that I have learned many things through New Direction, from Sarah and Bruce and Sue Jeep, the dietician.

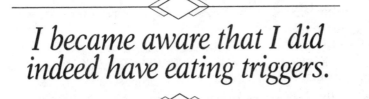

I became aware that I did indeed have eating triggers.

I knew going in what some of my problems were, at least on the surface. I ate too much. I ate much too fast. And hunger was nearly irrelevant. When we talked about behavior modification, I tried to imagine myself disciplined, thoughtful, controlled, with food in its proper perspective. It is fuel, it is medicinal, and isn't it nice that it's also pleasurable and tasty. Anyone can wait a few hours between meals and allow natural hunger to develop. I had no fear of going without or, worse, starving.

I had the toughest time with the concept of eating triggers. I've never been aware of eating any more or less during times of stress, anxiety, pain, grief, excitement, happiness. My joke was that my trigger is the sun coming up in the morning. Even if the sky is cloudy, I know the sun is up there somewhere. I never needed a reason to eat or to overeat. I did it because I just liked to eat. How many times have you heard or said that? "I just love food." Most people, even civilians, do.

So did I have no triggers, or was I simply unaware of them?

I learned a few things about myself during the modified fast portion of the program. After getting through the uncomfortable initial stages, I was impressed and intrigued with the lack of physical hunger. It is true that I rarely felt real hunger in the past because I was always eating or recuperating from eating. But to literally not eat solids and still not feel hunger was fascinating. Of course, I was glad about it.

I yearned to eat, and I longed to have a meal, but not because my stomach was empty or growling. I did notice, however, that besides the media reminders of food (commercials, jingles, pictures, logos) and the smells from the kitchen, there were other times when I missed food more intensely. And, *voilà*, those were emotional times.

I have always considered myself a very even person emotionally. If anything, I am more sentimental and perhaps romantic than the average adult male. I am one who can be moved to tears more easily than most. I am nostalgic. I rarely show my anger, and even my family would admit that I probably haven't raised my voice half a dozen times in two decades.

Does that mean I bury my true feelings? Do I eat them away rather than expose and deal with them? I'm an optimist, usually up, but not too far up. Is my every emotion anesthetized by food? I never thought so. But on the modified fast, I did notice that a slight, an insult, a disappointment triggered something. And my first thought was food.

Now this was a very difficult, traumatic time, as you can imagine. I can't overemphasize how quickly I might have failed had I also had to deal with real hunger. Yet, still, this was a battle of endurance over temptation. I was succeeding and I was gratified with my accomplishment. It rocked me to notice that certain setbacks I had hardly been aware of in the past now made me think how much I missed food and how nice it would be to be able to head for the refrigerator.

Sometimes I even did that, not to cheat (I assume I've made that point sufficiently) but to chow down on some diet Jell-O or fill up on water or diet drinks. I still felt as if I was overeating. In a way, I was. Though I was still within the program and was not consuming enough to slow my five-pounds-a-week loss, I felt less control. And I became aware that I did indeed have eating triggers.

Another trigger was at the other end of the emotional scale. When I heard good news, accomplished something, received a compliment, any affirmation, I had the same feeling: I wanted to eat, I suppose to celebrate. The negative trigger was stronger and more likely to result in consumption, but the positive trigger was real too. I would not have learned those things about myself without being restricted to an all-liquid diet for those seventeen weeks.

I have also learned about a very disappointing trigger. With all the classes I have sat through and the good input I've heard from Sarah and Sue and other leaders—and also from fellow strugglers—I have heard about many, many triggers. Some of those I could identify with. People talked about smells, sights, sounds, situations, locations that all contributed to the desire to overeat. I kept looking for my triggers.

Was my trigger a buffet situation? I've learned to avoid those or to eat in advance and refrain. (I often succeed in party situations by subtly letting it be known that I'm simply not eating anything during that time. It doesn't create a ruckus, and then I'm not worried who's watching or counting crackers or judging my piece of cake.)

Was my trigger a lag time in the afternoon between work and dinner, as many people said? Many talked about doing well until those afternoon doldrums when they just started snacking and couldn't stop. No, for me it wasn't that.

Neither was my trigger late-night snacking, which I had done without thinking in the past.

Other people said their triggers were normal eating times. Hungry or not, if the clock said it was lunchtime, it was lunchtime.

Sometimes just being in the car makes buzzing into a drive-through irresistible. Being in a movie theater and smelling popcorn triggered others.

What was it that made me overeat now? How disappointing to discover that my food trigger is—are you ready?—food.

Bummer.

I can be doing well, staying within my calorie counts and fat percentages, enjoying my frozen yogurt treats as harmless fillers. Then, if I don't get busy with something else and let that mechanism in my stomach tell my brain I've had enough, I can justify all kinds of things. I can have the perfect lunch for my program and then want to buzz into a drive-through fast-food place for another cone or two.

Don't get me wrong. My program can probably handle it. But once I am outside my calorie counts I can get discouraged and not look forward to making all the necessary adjustments. Do I really want to cut dinner in half now because I overdid it on the way home from lunch? Or, just like the poisonous thinking from the past, do I want to blow off today and start fresh tomorrow?

That is the most dangerous thinking of all, of course, but it has been one of the toughest for me to overcome. Often I don't overcome it. I may be only a few hundred calories over my limit by midday and still have every chance of succeeding for the day, but, if I don't rein myself in quickly, I can unravel. What was a bit of an aberration but still well within my program can suddenly be rationalized into a blown day that can include all manner of bingeing.

I have also learned why we binge, and it came from someone else in one of the classes. He said, "We eat like there's no tomorrow because we tell ourselves, 'I can never do this again. This is the last time I will ever binge, so I have to have everything I want.'"

I used to think that my satiety mechanism (that stomach-to-brain message that says I've had enough) was slow because I ate so fast. That was true, of course, but I have also come to learn that I subconsciously have made myself eat fast to stay ahead of that mechanism. I see the amount of food I want, and I know if I eat slowly I'll get full too soon and won't be able to have it all. Ugly, isn't it?

I confess that the one area I have not succeeded in is slowing down. I've tried all the tricks. Chewing more. Counting bites and chews. Putting my fork down between bites. Leaving some food on purpose. Saving half the meal till later. Telling myself that if I'm still hungry in twenty minutes I can have more. (That one comes closest to working for me, by the way. When food has triggered the desire for more food and I am psyched in and committed to not overeating, I'll tell myself, "Wait twenty minutes and you can have whatever you want." By then my pseudo hunger is usually gone, and I'm home free.)

I find that I do best when I plan ahead, allocate my food specifically, and tell myself in advance that, though food triggers in me a phony hunger or need to eat more, I will stop and wait when I'm finished with my allotted meal. Then I have to get out of the kitchen or off the road. I have even driven circuitous routes to avoid tempting fast-food places.

Understand, I have kicked the cheeseburger habit, though I know I would still love those. Some things (like Quarter Pounders) simply have to be put aside forever and substituted with other things (like McLeans). What I'm talking about avoiding are those things that would otherwise be fine on my program —like more low-fat, or even no-fat, yogurt cones. I am living proof that merely keeping your fat percentages down is not enough. I, like most people, can consume more than enough low-fat calories and still gain weight.

Probably the biggest handicap I now face is that I can rarely eat with my own family. Fortunately I work largely at home and am diligent in carving out time with the family. But one of my major weaknesses is unlimited supplies of food. While Dianna cooks good, healthy, balanced meals, they are higher in fat than what I should have. And I have learned enough about myself to know that I will find a way to justify finishing the serving bowl or having one, two, or three extra helpings of something that otherwise would be fine.

Sometimes, when we carefully plan ahead, I prepare my own meal and sit with the family. This works best the day or two before my weekly weigh-in when, yes, I am stronger. I hate to admit about myself that I am too weak in "family serving" situations to succeed, but I have to go with what works. I succeed much better when we occasionally eat out together.

Most distasteful and yet probably most helpful about what I've learned is in the area of lapsing, recovering, and why the battle still rages despite all we know and all we have accomplished. And that is next.

24

Hard Truth, Part 1:
Calling a Spade a Spade

I used to take great comfort in comparing myself to other fat people. I was often the heaviest person in any setting I found myself—and that is still mostly true—but I rarely looked it. Sure, you see the picture on the back of this book, and yes, I was one of those huge people who draws stares and makes everyone else feel trim.

But I carried my weight differently than most who weigh that much. I bought clothes that were big enough to actually leave me room. I was not comfortable in that body, of course, but I was comfortable in my clothes. I never understood heavy people who added the burden of tight-fitting clothes to their problems. Perhaps they didn't have the means to buy larger clothes as they got heavier, but I've also seen people try to tell themselves that they haven't really graduated to a bigger size.

I once saw a man scowl as he tried on a suit he could barely button. "I'd better try the 50," he muttered.

"That *is* a 50," the salesperson said.

The man was so disgusted with himself that he bought the 50!

I know that allowing ourselves to admit that we have moved up a size makes it seem as if we are giving ourselves license to quit being ever vigilant about our food and our diets.

Frankly, however, when I was suffering and trying to get a handle on my problem, I needed the breather of not also worrying about tight clothes. Maybe to some people tight clothes are motivation to eat less. For me the discomfort would have irrationally made me feel I deserved something good to eat.

Something else I recommend, especially (but not exclusively) to men: wear your belt at, not below, your waist. Yes, it causes a bit more discomfort when seated, and if you are unusually large your abdomen may protrude. But that is a small trade-off for how you look when standing and walking with your belt tucked up under your belly. That's one of the looks that gives big people a bad name. Burying the belt, buckle and all, and letting your stomach hang over makes it appear that you are giving room to the expanse and are perhaps planning to expand some more.

While you're working on a solution to your problem, buy pants and belts big enough to go around you; pull those pants up, and buy a coat you can button comfortably. You'll feel better and look better. You won't look and feel as good as you can—and will—when you lose your weight and start maintaining it, but you'll sure look and feel better than when you are squeezed into your clothes.

I can't pretend to speak for women, but I have always appreciated those larger women who don't try to pretend that they are a couple of sizes smaller than they are. This society is even crueler to women than to us men, and there will be snide comments regardless of what you wear. But clearly you appear more comfortable and at ease with yourself when you wear clothes that give you room to move and breathe.

Another comparison that used to make me feel good about myself—misguided though I was—was that I didn't have binge stories. Now, you may remember my out-of-control days when I was frequenting the fast-food places and gorging on big, greasy sandwiches several times a day, and you say, "That wasn't bingeing?"

In a way, it wasn't. I was on a certain regimen. I was eating so much that I probably didn't have room to binge even if I had wanted to. "Wanted to" is the wrong term, of course. Bingers feel *compelled*; it would be inaccurate to say they "want to" binge.

I was always fascinated by people who told stories about eating half a jar of mayonnaise right from the refrigerator. Or a whole two-pound bag of M&Ms. Or an entire box of chocolates. For some strange reason, I allowed myself to mentally distance myself from those "real" problem eaters because that was something I never did.

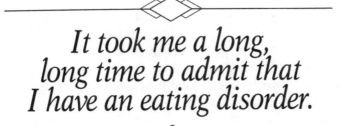

It took me a long, long time to admit that I have an eating disorder.

I never binged and purged. I was never anorexic. I allowed for the possibility that I was a compulsive overeater. But I avoided the term "eating disorder" like the plague. To me that sounded like a cop-out. People who were bulimic or anorexic had eating disorders. I, and other heavy people like me, was just an undisciplined or compulsive overeater. I believed that unless someone had been diagnosed by a psychiatrist, he or she used the eating disorder line as an excuse. And so I avoided it.

It took me a long, long time to admit that I have an eating disorder. I do not use it as an excuse. I don't even claim that it is something I didn't bring on myself. But when a person does something he truly doesn't want to do, something he knows he will regret, he has a disorder.

I succeed when I plan ahead and allot myself certain portions of food. Because I still weigh well over 200 pounds, I am allowed a lot more calories per day than the average person— and certainly a lot more calories than the average fellow struggler. So I'm not starving. I'm rarely actually hungry. I am not deprived.

I am in the neighborhood of 130 pounds lighter than I was at my peak weight, and at this writing I have been maintaining that loss for more than a year and a half. I have learned about vitamins and nutrients, about fats, carbohydrates, and protein. I know things about sugar and salt and cholesterol and fiber that make me an obnoxious obsessive about food labeling. What can I say? I've become a shirtsleeve expert at weight loss and control.

BUT!

But I still struggle. I still fail. I have every motivation in the world to continue to succeed, and yet the battle rages. It doesn't get easier; it gets harder. I have total sympathy for those 96 out of 100 people who lose more than a hundred pounds and gain it back within a few years. I know exactly what they go through.

When well-meaning friends say, "Now what you need to do is keep it off," you want to scream, "No kidding, Sherlock! What a concept!"

When people say, "My aunt died on a diet like that. Are you sure it's healthy?" you want to say, "No, 'healthy' was weighing 380 and having diabetes!"

Who had more motivation than Oprah Winfrey, who lost all her weight and then had to face a network TV camera every day as the pounds came back on? Regardless of what she says or does about it, you can imagine the pain, the humiliation, the embarrassment.

I have never been a fan of Hollywood, and I think too many movie actors and actresses make a mockery of marriage and love. Yet even someone who has been married many times and has appeared in productions that should make Christians cringe does not deserve the type of treatment Elizabeth Taylor has received from the press and the public over the years.

One magazine featured celebrities who have waged the weight wars, including Delta Burke and Oprah and singer Luther Vandross and others. Along the top of the pages throughout the entire feature were photos of Liz Taylor through the last several decades, fat, then thin, then fat, then thin, and so on.

Who deserves that?

A snotty gossip column in a daily Chicago newspaper often announces where its correspondents have spotted Oprah or the mayor or anyone else chowing down. They tell what the celebrity ate and how many helpings. Yet one of the columnists is herself overweight. It's senseless.

But that's how society treats fat people, and so we have all the motivation we need to lose weight and keep it off. And yet we find it nearly impossible. The odds are against us. What is the problem? What is our eating disorder?

Civilians will tell you it's lack of discipline. Laziness. Stupidity. (As if we don't know how we got fat or what to do about it.) Many of us take comfort when we read that some people are predisposed to fat by heredity. Though there is truth to that, we sabotage ourselves by using it as an excuse. It may be a reason, and an unfair one at that, that we have to battle this condition all our lives, but it is no reason to resign ourselves to failure.

I've seen books by people who have lost prodigious amounts of weight, gleefully showing off their new look and offering advice on how to do it (sounds familiar). But then a year or two later, when the weight is back, they bring out another book about how the re-gain was inevitable and that they are actually healthier now. I don't want to be insensitive, and, as I said above, I am totally sympathetic to those in the battle. I know and fight the terrible odds against success. But the fact is that, whatever the reason we can't succeed, when we fail it's because we're consuming more calories than we are burning. Anyone who tells you that he or she gains weight under any other formula is a liar or a freak of nature.

Anyone with a weight problem can easily resent someone who seems to be able to eat whatever he or she wants and never gain weight. Worse is when they complain, "I'm having trouble keeping my weight up." Cry me a river.

Then there are those to whom food is almost meaningless. They have to remind themselves to eat. They feel a hunger pang late in the afternoon, smack themselves in the forehead and say, "That's right, I forgot lunch!" I don't know about you, but I have never forgotten a meal in my life.

So what is my eating disorder—the one I refuse to use as an excuse? I'm not sure what to call it, but it takes many forms. As I've said, I have to plan ahead and allot myself a certain amount of food, and then do something else until the "hunger" that food triggered subsides. I also know that I cannot leave food that I enjoy. I try to avoid pizza parties where I know there will be leftovers. I know how much I can have, and I may start with the best intentions. After taking my allowed number of slices and enjoying them, I'm headed for disaster if someone has left half a pizza sitting there.

Picnics, buffets, unlimited supplies—I've learned these are all dangerous for me. Also, being in situations where no one knows I have a weight problem or an eating problem can create hardship for me. Much as I resent it, I am more careful in public when people are around who know my history. They may not be watching or even thinking about it, but in my mind I am being judged by everything I put in my mouth. If I know no one knows or cares, I don't limit myself for any social reasons. Danger.

Why can't I leave food? I may never know. Had I been raised in poverty and had to fight for every serving, I would understand. I grew up with brothers, and, yes, if I didn't stab that pork chop as soon as I looked up from grace, I might get less than someone else. And in high school we had about twenty minutes for lunch, so we learned to eat quickly.

But I never went hungry. I have no history of missing a meal. When I was overweight, I thought about eating all the time. When I was fasting and losing weight, I thought about eating all the time. Now that I am maintaining, and succeeding, it still seems my day revolves around mealtimes, plans, food diaries, the scale. While I used to consider myself emotionally even, now I find myself up and down depending on what the scale says or how I am succeeding or failing in keeping control of my totals and percentages. It's not a fun way to live, but when I compare myself (here I go again) with people who really suffer and struggle throughout the world, I realize I have a pretty minor problem in the global scheme.

What puzzled me most and dominated my thinking the longest was the psychological aspect of all of this. The heredity is there, the predisposition to weight, the body style, the body chemistry, the formerly active but now mostly sedentary lifestyle—all are excuses I could use. And yet I lost and have maintained. The question is why is it still so hard? Why hasn't it gotten easier? Why can't I just "change my lifestyle?"

I have as much motivation as anyone. I have a young family. I have pride and ego. I am writing this book with my "before and after" pictures on the back cover. I am diabetic, but need no medication as long as the weight stays down. Civilians are not the only ones who wonder why it shouldn't be logical and simple to simply do it. Stay down. Stay at it. Keep up the good work.

By all manner of reckoning, I should never overeat again. I should be able to overcome any temptation. I know my weaknesses. I know my triggers. I know what could start me on the slippery slope of failure.

And yet I continue to battle this monster every day, this eating disorder or whatever you will allow me to call it. I have the knowledge, the program, the techniques, the tools, and above all, the motivation. But I still have my failures and my setbacks.

If you are a Christian, this should start sounding familiar to you. You may have been afraid that I would start coming to an uncomfortable conclusion. Will I, of all people, hint that a person's painful struggle in the area of weight control has something to do with personal, moral failure? While civilians are accusing us of being selfish, lazy, undisciplined, and not caring, will I, one of our own number, say that our problem is the result of sin? Are we gluttons? And if I say that, will it help anyone?

25

Hard Truth, Part 2: Romans 7 Personified

I confess to sneaking up on you with the more biblical spiritual aspect to this story. The reason has as much to do with me as with you. If indeed we are fellow strugglers, then I can write to you only the way I would want to be written to. I'm afraid I would not pick up a book that told me I was a fat, compulsive overeater because I was a sinner. Other people are sinners too, but they do not wage this same war.

You may be wishing, and asking, "Can't we separate this medical, physical, psychological, problem of ours from biblical things? Can't we put it in the nail-biting category? Sure, it's more serious and life-threatening, but does everything have to be spiritual?

My answer may surprise you. My life, my calling, my work has been in Christian writing for the better part of my life, and yet I would say, no—even for the Christian, not everything has to be spiritual. There are those deeper and more educated than I who would disagree with me on that. And because they are deeper and more educated, I would not care to debate the issue with them.

But I believe there are life issues that can be dealt with somewhat separate from one's faith, though "he who is spiritual judges all things" (1 Corinthians 2:15). Paul says that "the natural man does not receive the things of the Spirit of God, for they are foolishness to him; nor can he know them, because they are spiritually discerned" (verse 14).

You may wonder why I want to make this very fleshly, very personal problem a spiritual matter. The fact is, I don't. I would rather relegate it to some neutral area where I could deal with it apart from the church, apart from my faith, apart from God. We each have our own peccadilloes, so let me have mine.

And yet I cannot. Oh, I tried. Like anyone else who has struggled and failed in this area, I prayed for strength. But when I failed again, could I blame God? Had He not answered my prayer? Was He not sufficient? Were His mercies not new every morning? Was there not a way of escape so that I could bear any temptation that has overtaken me?

I never thought God didn't care, of course. It was just that this was something I wished to compartmentalize, to separate from the spiritual. I didn't think about it consciously, which makes me think now that perhaps I was hiding from God on the issue in much the same way that Adam hid in the garden because of his shame. If I allowed this to be a spiritual matter, I would have to come to dark conclusions about myself. I didn't think, at first, that bringing God into His rightful place in even this ugly, seemingly peripheral area of my life would also open to me His infinite resources.

So I suggest to you that if fat and weight and the scale and diets have become your life, there is no alternative but to include God in the issue. We don't want to. This isn't murder. This isn't adultery. This isn't theft. We don't smoke or drink or chase. Nearly half the people in our churches are somewhat overweight. Isn't there room for one unmentioned, sort of dignified (you don't hassle me and I won't hassle you) evangelical weakness/mistake/aberration/glitch that doesn't have to be labeled out-and-out sin? Aren't there enough people accusing us of being weak slobs without our now worrying that God is scowling at us?

Well, of course He's not. He loves us. But much as I wanted to avoid the issue, what drove me to it was my desperation to get to the bottom of the whys. Why? Why? Why?

Why can people be so successful in many other difficult areas of their lives and not be able to gain the victory in this one?

Why can I overcome other bad habits and not get a handle on this one?

Why is it that, with all the motivation a person could ever want, I continue to struggle as a compulsive overeater, having to work out hard an hour a day, six days a week, keeping track by computer of everything I eat, and still occasionally find myself failing?

The people at New Direction are no doubt tired of hearing me harp, week after week, about the puzzling, aggravating psychological part of this. We know all the answers, the reasons, the techniques, the hints, the tricks, the consequences of lapsing, and yet we lapse anyway. We tell ourselves we don't want to overeat, to binge, to fall off the wagon. We even know full well and tell ourselves we'll regret our actions. If we eat this, when we're not hungry, when we don't need it, when we've done so well, we will feel bad about ourselves, we will feel guilty, we will regret it. And then we do it anyway and all those things become true.

Have you—like me—had those times where you get it into your head that you are going to cheat, to overeat, to go off your program, to have what you want when you want it? You know every reason not to and you know it goes against all sense and wisdom. You know you'll regret it and pay for it and may even hate yourself for it. But you do it anyway.

Our weight war is Romans 7 personified.

Aside from sin, selfishness, gluttony, instant self-gratification, looking out for number one, it makes no sense. Why are we self-destructive? Some of us have reasons—maybe not good ones, but understandable ones. Maybe we were abused as children, neglected, whatever. Maybe our families were dysfunctional, and try as we might we can't live in reaction to that but rather under the circumstances of that. We are repeating our parents' mistakes rather than correcting them.

But what about those of us who can't point to such baggage? What makes a person like me, with absolutely everything in the world going for him, do things I don't want to do? What makes me do things I know I will regret? What makes me make life harder on myself, forcing me to have to compensate for failures just to stay even?

When I told myself every day of that torturous seventeen-week modified fast that that was the easy part and that keeping the weight off would be the hard part, but that I would never give up, why do I still find myself on the edge of self-destruction nearly every week? It makes no sense. At least apart from Scripture it makes no sense.

I hate to think of myself as a carnal man. I have been a Christian most of my life. I have not been as consistent and devout and disciplined as I would like, but I want to serve God and love Him more. I want to do what is right. I believe I have a handle on personal salvation, knowing that in me dwells no good thing and that my only hope of heaven rests in the work Jesus did on my behalf.

So why must I continue to live with this battle between the old and the new natures? Why do I still sin?

I don't know why, but I know I am not alone. I take great comfort in the fact that the Christian life is made up of a series of new beginnings. And as dark and ugly as are these revelations about myself, there is a glimmer of hope in the truth that the apostle Paul himself faced the same dilemma.

If you're a New Testament person, you know what I am talking about. From the pages of Romans 7 come the desperate, haunting, frustrating cries of the soul of one of the greatest evangelists the world has ever known. Paul was redeemed by Christ, and his life became dedicated to bringing others to God. And yet his agony resounds through the ages from the pages of Scripture, from the letter he wrote to the church in Rome.

If you're one of those who makes a habit of skipping over the Scripture references in an otherwise popular-level book like this, do me a favor and read these verses anyway. You have stayed with me this far, so hear me out. If you are a fellow struggler, you can apply the sentiments from this passage to our common problem. It may seem nearly sacrilegious to apply Paul's heart-cry to an eating problem, and I'm not suggesting that compulsive overeating was his thorn in the flesh. But you may be as struck as I have been that our weight war is Romans 7 personified.

Paul writes in Romans 7:15–25:

> For what I am doing, I do not understand. For what I will to do, that I do not practice; but what I hate, that I do. If, then, I do what I will not to do, I agree with the law that it is good. Now then, it is no longer I who do it, but sin that dwells in me. For I know that in me (that is, in my flesh) nothing good dwells; for to will is present with me, but how to perform what is good I do not find. For the good that I will to do, I do not do; but the evil I will not to do, that I practice. Now if I do what I will not to do, it is no longer I who do it, but sin that dwells in me. I find then a law, that evil is present with me, the one who wills to do good. For I delight in the law of God according to the inward man. But I see another law in my members, warring against the law of my mind, and bringing me into captivity to the law of sin which is in my members. O wretched man that I am! Who will deliver me from this body of death? I thank God—through Jesus Christ our Lord! So then, with the mind I myself serve the law of God, but with the flesh the law of sin.

If you can identify, as I can, with the first part of that passage, you may be tempted to say—as many have said about any sin—"It's not me; it's the sin that dwells in me." That's a reason, but not an excuse. As Paul says in the same letter, "Shall we continue in sin that grace may abound? Certainly not!" (6:1–2).

But do you find as I do at least some comfort in the fact that we are not weird or unique? When you despair because of your inability to stay with the program, when you edge toward self-loathing because of your weakness, when you can't make sense of your weakness when you know better, remember that there is victory in the end. Who shall deliver us from the body of this death? With Paul we can thank God through Jesus Christ our Lord:

> There is therefore now no condemnation to those who are in Christ Jesus, who do not walk according to the flesh, but according to the Spirit. For the law of the Spirit of life in Christ Jesus has made me free from the law of sin and death. For what the law could not do in that it was weak through the flesh, God did by sending His own Son in the likeness of sinful flesh and for sin, condemned sin in the flesh, that the righteous requirement of the law might be fulfilled in us who do not walk according to the flesh but according to the Spirit. . . . But if the Spirit of Him who raised Jesus from the dead dwells in you, He who raised Christ from the dead will also give life to your mortal bodies through His Spirit who dwells in you. Therefore, brethren, we are debtors not to the flesh, to live according to the flesh. For if you live according to the flesh you will die; but if you through the Spirit put to death the deeds of the body, you will live. For as many as are led by the Spirit of God, these are sons of God. . . . He who did not spare His own Son, but delivered Him up for us all, how shall He not with Him also freely give us all things? . . . Who shall separate us from the love of Christ? Shall tribulation, or distress, or persecution, or famine, or nakedness, or peril, or sword? As it is written: "For Your sake we are killed all day long; we are accounted as sheep for the slaughter." Yet in all these things we are more than conquerors through Him who loved us. For I am persuaded that neither death nor life, nor angels nor principalities nor powers, nor things present nor things to come, nor height nor depth, nor any other created thing, shall be able to separate us from the love of God which is in Christ Jesus our Lord. (Romans 8:1–4, 11–14, 32, 35–39)

Might a scholar or theologian accuse me of reaching for application here? Perhaps. Paul no doubt was not thinking of me and my weight wars when he penned those words. He was writing of the battle of the ages, Satan versus Christ, sin and death against righteousness and life. And yet I am affirmed when I read that the God who didn't spare His own Son for my sake would also freely give me all things. And who can fail to be moved by the litany of all those mighty things that are unable to separate us from the love of Christ?

If none of those can separate us, can our own weakness, our own compulsions, our own habits, our fat, our weight, our inconsistencies? Sin separated us, but Jesus, who knew no sin, became sin for us. And so now nothing can separate us. To know that my eternal destiny is set because of the work of Christ on my behalf frees me to quit trying to earn it.

And strangely, knowing that Paul and all my Christian ancestors battled the powers of sin and darkness in their own bodies and despaired over their inability to do "the good that I will to do," doesn't cause me to give up. I don't simply resign myself to the human condition. I thank God through Jesus Christ that the victory can be mine.

The battle still rages, but now I can determine to never give up, to always start over, to stop taking one step forward and two steps back. I have learned that I will rarely take two steps forward without at least one step back, but I have been freed from perfectionism. I have been loosed from the bondage of "proving" to myself that I can't succeed.

I know I can't succeed in the flesh, so I put my faith in the Christ of Calvary. He will continue to forgive and to empower me to stay in the war. I might have wished that He could miraculously deliver me from my sin and weakness and cravings and failure. But that is not how life is in any area this side of heaven.

If you can find your way clear of the myth of a sudden change to sinless perfection—with your weight or with any other shortcoming in your life—you will find yourself energized to stay at the task and able to make use of the advice I close with in the final chapter.

26

Where to Go from Here

If you have permitted me to apply some of the wonderful truths of the New Testament to our common problem, you must go a bit further and enjoy all the benefits. I told you from the beginning that I had no magic formulas, no surefire guarantees that you would never again fail. All I offered was sympathy and hints from my own experience.

But no matter where you are on your journey—getting ready to lose a significant amount, trying to maintain a loss, or despairing over having put back weight you lost—you should enjoy applying some of the great Scripture passages to your experience. If it is true that the core of our problem is self and sin, consider how freeing and exciting are the following passages.

"If we confess our sins, He is faithful and just to forgive us our sins and to cleanse us from all unrighteousness" (1 John 1:9). That is one of the most well-known and popular verses in the New Testament, with good reason. We all want to know that forgiveness is there for us, because we are so maddeningly consistent in our weakness and our humanness.

Psalm 32:1–7 says,

> Blessed is he whose transgression is forgiven, whose sin is covered. Blessed is the man to whom the Lord does not impute in-

iquity, and in whose spirit there is no guile. When I kept silent, my bones grew old through my groaning all the day long. For day and night Your hand was heavy upon me; my vitality was turned into the drought of summer. I acknowledged my sin to You, and my iniquity I have not hidden. I said, "I will confess my transgressions to the Lord," and You forgave the iniquity of my sin. For this cause everyone who is godly shall pray to You in a time when You may be found; surely in a flood of great waters they shall not come near him. You are my hiding place; You shall preserve me from trouble; You shall surround me with songs of deliverance.

May we never be so old in the faith or so jaded that we cannot exult in that truth!

I was discussing my problem with a Christian friend, and I bounced off him the idea that I had concluded that it was sin, part of the human condition, and that Satan had attacked me in one of my weakest areas. Almost immediately he said, "If that's true, and you continue to be tempted, you should be pretty joyful all the time." I was stunned. Joyful is not what I would call it. Frustrated. Angry with myself. Sometimes despairing.

He continued, "If you're going to apply Scripture, you must apply all of Scripture." I was still listening. "James 1 says, 'Count it all joy when you fall into various trials, knowing that the testing of your faith produces patience'" (verses 2–3).

What a window that opened for me! I wanted my maintenance to become easier. I know more, I have more reasons to succeed, and yet still I find myself failing and having to start over. For this I am to count it all joy. I am to be happy because the testing of my faith produces patience!

Even better than that, a few verses later James says, "Blessed is the man who endures temptation; for when he has been proved, he will receive the crown of life which the Lord has promised to those who love Him" (James 1:12).

I don't want to be unkind, but in the event that you feel I've copped out or overspiritualized this issue, let me encourage you to keep trying all the things you have tried over the years. If your experience is like mine, you will come to the end of yourself and your human efforts and will have to turn back to God.

So where does that leave us? I still have advice, things that have helped me. The above Scripture is there for you when you try your best to do it right and still find yourself failing. Count it all joy that you have been tempted, live in the Spirit to gain the victory, and, should you stumble, confess, repent, and get back in the battle.

Meanwhile, here are some very basic things that have been helpful to me—and may be to you:

1 Never skip breakfast, even if you overate the night before and don't feel hungry in the morning. It has been proven that people who eat breakfast gain less weight than those who don't, even if they may consume a few more calories. The breakfast gets your metabolism and your digestive system going.

2 Don't eat lunch until your body tells you it needs it. This is difficult, but you will enjoy your lunch more. If you feel the need to snack in between, make sure it's something that will fill you up and add bulk and fiber and that it is on your program. (Also, try drinking something noncaloric instead of snacking. You may have mistaken thirst for hunger.)

3 Don't allow yourself to get too hungry, because that leads to overeating. A hunger pang that cannot be satisfied with a glass of water or diet pop or coffee is a real one, and you should go ahead and have your lunch.

4 Plan ahead, keeping track not only of what you have eaten but of what you expect to eat. Learn (or use a guide) to keep track of calorie counts, fat percentages, and vitamins and nutrients. Maintaining the right calories and fat percentages can still leave you malnourished if you're not getting your United States Department of Agriculture recommended daily allowances (U.S. RDA) of vitamins and nutrients.

5 Double the fiber you're used to. Build slowly to this point. Fiber doesn't have to be distasteful but can come in the form of fruits and vegetables. To be sure, add a high fiber cereal to a drink or other snack.

6 Drink all the fluids you can handle, and then some. Anything noncaloric will benefit you, and avoiding caffeine is even better, because caffeine is a natural diuretic and can flush nutrients from your system.

7 Eat more frequently than you are used to, but give yourself permission. Plan ahead, allocate portions, stop when you're satisfied, and stay within your totals. Proper snacking can keep your blood sugar levels more consistent and help you avoid inappropriate hunger and overeating.

8 Avoid danger areas, such as routes past places you can't pass up without indulging.

9 Don't cut out any treat entirely unless you know it throws you off and you know you can stay away from it forever. Better to enjoy a little and work it in to keep from bingeing.

10 Tell someone who will love and support you exactly what you are doing. Even if you don't give him permission to nag or remind you, simply telling him, "I'm going to this party, and I am not going to have any nuts or ice cream," will help you follow through, even if they are not there. I have told friends that I was going to lose—or not gain—on certain trips and found that that promise alone has kept me on course.

11 Make dinner your last meal of the day, unless you have a medical condition that requires a midevening snack. This has been crucial for me, and I do best on my program when I follow it. If I can get past seven or eight o'clock in the evening, I can generally talk myself out of ruining the day with something additional to eat. I miss out on some fun things, such as snacking in front of the TV or having a late-night dessert, but I always feel better in the morning and am hungry for breakfast.

12 Chart your weight on a graph and look at it regularly. When I don't do this, I am stunned at the inevitable drift. When I have a graphic reminder, I am motivated to stay at the task. (This requires regular weigh-ins, preferably weekly, on a dependable scale.)

13 Don't be afraid of a reward system. If you are like me, getting started on the wrong foot can ruin the whole day. I start justifying things or working extras into my pro-

gram, telling myself I will adjust later meals to compensate. By midafternoon I'm at my calorie count for the whole day and know I shouldn't skip dinner altogether. You know what happens next. The old lies about, "Well, since I've already shot this day, I might as well have . . ." begin in my mind and I justify all manner of horrible things. That leads to remorse, regret, depression, feelings of failure, temptations to give up.

Rather, reward yourself for passing up certain things. Allow yourself a special treat if you make it to lunch without snacking. Make sure it's a treat that fits what you're trying to accomplish and doesn't throw you off. There are those who would say that looking at food as a reward is part of our problem, but I say it's also realistic. We do love food, and we associate it with happy memories. There can be more such memories if we get control of our intake.

14 Begin an exercise program slowly and keep working up until you can be healthy and vigorous and look forward to your almost-every-day heart workout. Invest in the right clothes and equipment or memberships and do it right. You'll become addicted to health.

15 Never give up. You will be tempted to. You will despair. You'll have lapses and relapses. You'll get back on that bike or in that water or on that walk and realize that you allowed yourself to get out of shape and wonder what's the use? But anything you do to get back on track is good, even if you have to make up for lost ground.

No one said you had to be perfect. No one said you had to work out every day. The more the better, and the sooner you get back to it, the easier it will be.

If I have learned or taken nothing else from the program I've been on, I have benefited from realizing that there is no end to the battle. I make no guarantees or promises. I am no more confident of long-term success today than I was two years ago today (at this writing) when I started New Direction. I am, however, committed and determined to stay at it. It seems that everything in my mind and body works against me. I am getting older. My bad habits are still in my mind. My body has that maddening set point that is usually fifty pounds more than what I weigh, and it continues to try to get me to eat enough and work out as little as it takes to get there.

My body wants to store fat. My brain tells me I'm hungry when I'm not. It also tells me I still need food, long after I have eaten enough to be satisfied. I want to be trim and lean and firm, and yet part of me wants to be full and fat.

And so I will simply say this: I am staying in the battle. I urge you to join it and stay in as well. I can do nothing about insensitive people who say the wrong things or who sabotage my efforts. I can do little about my own humanness and sinfulness and selfishness.

I can see my weakness and my sin only for what it is, count it all joy when I am tempted, rest in the work of Christ to deliver me, and be eternally grateful that I can "keep on continuing" to start over as many times as I need to.

It is only when I look back on these two very brief years that I realize, in spite of how long and hard the journey has been, that I have seen tremendous progress. I lost more and kept it off longer than ever. Though I wish it had become easier and not harder, I am confident only that God will give me the wherewithal to stay at it.

If this has been of any help to you, I'd love to hear from you and be able to pray for you by name. And I would be most grateful to know that you have done the same for me.